The Treatment of
Hypertension

CURRENT STATUS OF MODERN THERAPY: VOLUME 1

The Treatment of
Hypertension

Edited by

E.D. Freis

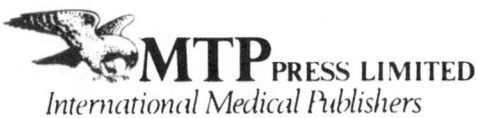

MTPPRESS LIMITED
International Medical Publishers

Published by
MTP Press Limited
Falcon House
LANCASTER, England

ISBN 978-94-015-7137-1   ISBN 978-94-015-7135-7 (eBook)
DOI 10.1007/978-94-015-7135-7

Contents

List of Contributors

F. A. FINNERTY, JR, MD
  Director, Hypertension Center of Washington, DC,
  1341Pennsylvania Avenue, S.E., Washington, DC 20003; Clinical
  Professor of Medicine, George Washington University School of
  Medicine, Washington, DC 20037, USA

E. D. FREIS, MD
  Senior Medical Investigator, Veterans Administration Hospital and
  Professor of Medicine, Georgetown University School of Medicine,
  Washington, DC 20422, USA

R. W. GIFFORD JR, MD
  Head, Department of Hypertension and Nephrology,
  The Cleveland Clinic Foundation, 9500 Euclid Avenue, Cleveland,
  OH 44106, USA

M. D. GUAZZI, MD
  Istituto Ricerche Cardiovasculari and Centro Ricerche
  Cardiovasculari del CNR, Via Francesco Sforza, 35, 20122 Milan,
  Italy

P. LUND-JOHANSEN, MD
  Professor in Medicine, University of Bergen School of Medicine,
  Medical Department A, 5016 Haukeland Hospital, Bergen,
  Norway

M. MOSER, MD
  Clinical Professor of Medicine, New York Medical College,
  Valhalla, New York; Physician in Charge, Hypertension Section,
  Westchester County Medical Center; Senior Medical Consultant,
  National High Blood Pressure Education Program, National
  Institutes of Health

R. READER
  National Heart Foundation of Australia, PO Box 2, Woden,
  Canberra, ACT 2606 Australia

Consultant Editor's Note

Current Status of Modern Therapy

Series Editor: J. Marks, Girton College, Cambridge.

The *Current Status of Modern Therapy* is a major new series from MTP Press with the purpose of providing a definitive view of modern therapeutic practice in those areas of clinical medicine in which important changes are occurring. The series consists of monographs specially commissioned under the individual editorship of internationally recognized experts in their fields. Their selection of a panel of contributors from many countries ensures an international perspective on developments in therapy.

The series will aim to review the growth areas of clinical pharmacology and therapeutics in a systematic way. It will be a continuing series in which the same subject areas will be covered by revised editions as advances make this desirable.

The Treatment of Hypertension is an ideal first volume for this new series. Major advances have been made over the past few years in the management of hypertension. These have led to dramatically reduced death rates secondary to cardiovascular disease. This volume reviews in an entirely practical format the new ideas that constitute effective management of the hypertensive patient concentrating on the *proven* important developments.

Preface

In the past few years there has been a great upsurge of interest in the problem of essential hypertension. This has been stimulated by several comparatively recent advances, the most important being the demonstration that many if not most of the complications of hypertension can be prevented with adequate and effective medical treatment. Because of the extremely high prevalence of hypertension (roughly one in six or seven adults) effective preventive treatment will have a tremendous impact on national health and longevity.

This new approach to the problem of hypertension differs markedly from the old, which concentrated on a meticulous and expensive search for curable forms of hypertension representing at most 5% of the hypertensive population. Today, however, we are facing up to a much greater challenge. Now many patients with hypertension, not just a selected fraction, are possible candidates for treatment. Therapeutic decisions need to be made which will affect the health and well-being of millions of people. This change has been truly revolutionary as, for the first time, it has become possible to influence a leading cardiovascular disorder therapeutically and prevent its complications.

This volume presents the current thought of leading experts in the new movement in hypertension. Their purpose is to supply the most recent information in the field in such a way that it can be applied by the physician in practice. In fact, this book is intended as a guide to the new management of hypertension.

Dr Ralph Reader introduces his subject by pointing out that the heightened interest in hypertension at present is the result of the convergence of several important developments occurring during the past 15–20 years. These included the US National Health Survey, which demonstrated the extremely high prevalence of hypertension, and the Framingham and other prospective studies which, like the life insurance statistics that preceded them, indicated a considerably increased risk of major cardiovascular complications, even with modest elevations of blood pressure. Most important has been the development of effective antihypertensive agents and the subsequent demonstration that the major complications of hypertension can be prevented in moderate and severe hypertension.

Dr Reader then presents a comprehensive and expert discussion of the components of community control programmes in hypertension. The section on taking the blood pressure and the importance of repeated measurements should be read by everyone connected with professional health care delivery. Dr Reader emphasizes the importance of the family physician in detecting hypertension, as well as organized screening programmes. He draws on his considerable experience in this area to give us sound advice on the costs of screening and the pitfalls to be avoided. Dr Reader concludes by discussing whether patients with mild hypertension should be treated; he concludes that the evidence is insufficient to make a sound judgment. He avoids making any therapeutic recommendations in this group of patients, which is perhaps a wiser course than I chose in my discussion of this subject.

In his description of the hypertensive work-up *Dr Ray Gifford* convincingly argues for a simple, basic examination that is both rapidly accomplished and relatively inexpensive. Drawing on his extensive experience at the Cleveland Clinic he describes useful clinical methods for screening for curable forms of hypertension and for evaluating the extent of target organ disease. Indications for special tests are spelled out. Dr Gifford presents a carefully reasoned programme for obtaining the optimal cost–benefit results from the examination of the hypertensive patient.

At first glance the task of managing hypertension appears to be one of tremendous proportions, because it is such a frequently encountered disorder. However, as I point out in my discussion of the effectiveness of treatment, the number of patients in whom treatment is definitely indicated is considerably less than the number diagnosed as being hypertensive on screening programmes. In fact, the diagnosis of chronic hypertension cannot legitimately be made on the basis of a single examination.

Blood pressure fluctuates widely even in normotensive persons, and is influenced by strong emotional reactions. A significant percentage of patients found to be hypertensive on the initial screening examination (as high as 50% in one survey) will revert to normotension on repeated testing and will, therefore, be eliminated as candidates for treatment. By far the greatest proportion of hypertensive patients who remain after eliminating these labile cases are in the mild classification. It is precisely in this large group of patients that the question of the effectiveness of drug treatment is most undecided. Should an intensive medical effort be made to enlist this vast group of mild cases into long-term treatment programmes? Or should they remain without treatment but under surveillance, so that the fraction who graduate to more severe grades of hypertension can quickly be detected and treated before they develop vascular complications? There are no immediate answers to these important questions which affect the lives of millions of people. My discussion is based on the evidence obtained from the controlled therapeutic trials that have been completed to date. Based on these findings I have attempted to set up certain guidelines for selecting patients with mild hypertension for treatment. These guidelines will be considered too conservative by some and too interventionist by others, depending on how the reader interprets the available information which, unfortunately, is still incomplete with respect to mild hypertension.

Dr Per Lund-Johansen has had a very extensive experience in assessing the haemodynamic effects of many hypotensive agents. He is, therefore, well qualified to describe how the various antihypertensive agents lower blood pressure in man. He also presents the mode of action, haemodynamic effects, absorption and excretion and side-effects of these agents. New drugs such as prazosin and minoxidil are also covered, and the rational use of drug combinations is presented.

Dr Marvin Moser describes the treatment of essential hypertension from the viewpoint of his own extensive clinical experience. All modalities of medical treatment, including low-salt and weight-reducing diets, sedatives and even behavioural modification techniques are discussed. Dr Moser is well known for his role in developing the current recommendations of the Joint National Committee Report (US) on Detection, Evaluation and Treatment of High Blood Pressure. It is not surprising, therefore, that he follows these recommendations closely. He also discusses the more important side-effects of the most-used antihypertensive agents, and emphasizes the important role the physician must play in obtaining good compliance.

Dr Maurizio Guazzi divides his discussion of the treatment of special forms of hypertension into three sections. The first section is devoted to hypertensive crisis, where immediate parenteral therapy is described using drugs such as diazoxide, sodium nitroprusside and trimethaphan. The indications and contraindications of the various drugs are ably presented in relation to the type of organ dysfunction present in the various types of hypertension, such as hypertension complicated by cerebrovascular insufficiency, angina, heart failure, etc.

In the second section Dr Guazzi takes up the subject of the toxaemias of pregnancy. He makes a sharp distinction between the hypertension that is associated with chronic renal disease or essential hypertension and pre-eclampsia and eclampsia which are uniquely associated with pregnancy. The latter remains a challenging and elusive pathogenic and therapeutic syndrome. Antihypertensive drugs are of little value in this condition, and early delivery of the fetus still seems to be the most satisfactory approach.

The third section is concerned with the various forms of renal hypertension, including not only primary renal diseases such as glomerulonephritis but also end-stage renal disease, whether primary or secondary to nephrosclerosis. The discussion of renovascular hypertension reflects the conservatism that has arisen in recent years, in part as a result of disappointment with surgical therapy, in part due to the rarity of finding truly curable patients with renovascular hypertension, and in part to the increased recognition of the benefits of antihypertensive therapy.

The most difficult problem to deal with in the treatment of hypertensive patients is non-compliance. Because they feel well, and because the threat of complications may lie far in the future, patients often are poorly motivated to continue with treatment. This is particularly true when the drugs induce disturbing side-effects. *Dr Frank Finnerty*, who carried out pioneering studies in this area, was the first to point out how ill-suited hospital clinics are to the successful long-term management of patients with hypertension. The key to Dr Finnerty's approach is a close patient–therapist relationship, which he believes requires more time and attention than the average physician can afford to give. Therefore he feels that following diagnosis and initiation of treatment the long-term management should be turned over to a physician's assistant, nurse clinician or a specially trained paramedical person. These individuals should be specially trained to educate and motivate the patients. While non-compliance may be less of a problem in some practices than in others, it is indeed a common occurrence in most clinical settings. Dr Finnerty's ideas are, therefore, worthy of careful study.

Hypertension is a leading cause of death in most countries of the world. It is the most frequent cardiovascular condition seen in medical practice. Yet therapy is available which is effective in preventing complications. The most recent vital statistics in the United States disclosed a striking fall of 21% in mortality rates for hypertension and a 14% decline for hypertensive heart disease in the brief period from 1972 to 1975. It was in 1972 that large educational programmes, both for the public and for physicians, were mounted all over the country. If these striking declines in death-rates are, in fact, the result of better recognition and more effective treatment, we may look forward in the future to even greater falls in morbidity and mortality as the new appr oaches to hypertension become more widely adapted and aggressively practised by physicians everywhere.

EDWARD D. FREIS

Washington, DC
March 1978

1

How effective is the medical treatment of hypertension?

E. D. Freis

INTRODUCTION

Prevalence of hypertension

Approximately one in seven adults have hypertension. The extraordinary prevalence is based on the criterion of a diastolic blood pressure of 90 mmHg or more using the fifth phase of the Korotkoff sounds. Comparable prevalence is found in almost all sections of the world including Japan[1], Europe[2], Africa[3] and the United States[4]. The only exceptions are a few, scattered unacculturated societies in remote areas of the world where hypertension is rare or absent. This may be due to an absence of salt in the diet[5]. Aside from these rare exceptions, however, hypertension may truly be called an epidemic of worldwide proportions. It is the most frequent chronic disorder physicians everywhere meet in their practice.

Mortality from hypertension

While the danger of severe hypertension has always been recognized physicians have for years regarded diastolic readings below 100 or 110 mmHg as being of no pathological consequence. Indeed, the condition has been called 'benign' essential hypertension to emphasize the lack of pathological importance. However, prospective epidemiological studies[6,7] as well as life insurance statistics[8] have conclusively disproved the benign nature of essential hypertension. These studies show that, even with diastolic levels between 90 and 100 mmHg, the mortality rate over a 20-year period doubles as compared to normotensive subjects of the same age and sex. Furthermore, the risk increases markedly with each increment of blood pressure above this level.

Magnitude of the therapeutic problem

Since even modest elevations of blood pressure increase the risk of early

1

mortality some authors have recommended that all patients with hypertension receive life-long antihypertensive treatment. This recommendation implies that approximately one in approximately six adults will be treated ideally on a worldwide basis. However (as will be shown in the pages which follow) this extreme view neglects other important considerations which indicate a more selective approach to the treatment of hypertension. If the latter view is accepted, then the task of treating hypertension becomes one of more manageable proportions.

In order to gain a clearer perspective on the problem certain relevant aspects of hypertension need to be emphasized. They are as follows:

Distribution of hypertension by severity
The various grades of hypertension are not uniformly distributed. The prevalence is highest in the 90–95 mmHg group and drops progressively with increasing levels of blood pressure[9]. This means that the largest proportion of the hypertensive population is in the 90–105 mmHg range. If only a selected subset of this large group requires treatment the magnitude of the problem is considerably reduced.

True prevalence of hypertension
Almost all national surveys have based their statistics on a single encounter with the subjects. However, the results of recent screening programmes where the subjects with elevated readings are called back for a second or third examination have revealed the surprising fact that as many as 50% of those found to be hypertensive on the initial examination are normotensive on subsequent examinations[10]. Two important conclusions can be drawn from these re-screening programmes. The first is that single-encounter surveys grossly overestimate the prevalence of hypertension. The second is that a diagnosis of essential hypertension cannot be made from a single examination. It has been known for many years that emotions influence blood pressure and that the apprehension associated with the initial examination is sufficient to raise the blood pressure in otherwise normotensive individuals.

The physician seeing patients in private practice encounters the same problem. Often patients are in discomfort or are apprehensive because of some illness which brings them to the physician. Unless the blood pressure is extremely elevated the physician will do well to see the patient on several more occasions, and in an asymptomatic state, before deciding on the need for treatment.

Variable course of mild hypertension
The increased risk in mild hypertension is based on morbidity and

mortality data for large groups of such patients. Actually, the course of individual patients in the group is highly variable. Some revert to normal; the majority do not change significantly and some progress to a more severe stage[11]. There are no certain predictors of what course the patient will take, although there are helpful guides which will be described in a subsequent section. However, the only certain method is periodic re-examination of the patient.

Differing spectrum of complications in mild, moderate and severe hypertension

Mild hypertension is herein defined as an average diastolic blood pressure (average from three separate office or clinic visits) of 90–104 mmHg inclusive. Moderate hypertension includes the diastolic range of 105–114 mmHg and severe hypertension of 115 mmHg or higher. This classification utilizes the fifth phase of the Korotkoff sounds.

The spectrum of cardiovascular complications occurring in mild hypertension differs from that which occurs in more severe forms of hypertension. Hypertension aggravates and accelerates atherosclerosis, which accounts for the considerably increased incidence of myocardial infarction and atherothrombotic stroke in this disorder[12]. In mild hypertension the major complications are almost exclusively of the atherosclerotic type. In moderate hypertension atherosclerotic complications also occur, but such patients develop in addition other morbid events specifically related to hypertension. The latter include haemorrhagic strokes, congestive heart failure, renal failure, dissecting aortic aneurysm and the malignant phase of hypertension. Patients with severe hypertension usually do not live long enough to develop atherosclerotic complications unless their lives are prolonged by treatment. Otherwise, they generally succumb to one of the hypertensive complications.

Antihypertensive treatment is primarily effective against hypertensive complications. As will be shown later in this chapter the evidence to date fails to indicate any significant protection against atherosclerotic complications, particularly those involving the coronary arteries which are the most common type. It cannot be assumed, therefore, that if treatment is effective in reducing morbidity and mortality in moderate and severe hypertension it will be equally efficacious in mild hypertension. Nor does it follow that the excess mortality, which is due to atherosclerotic complications, can be significantly reduced by normalizing the blood pressure. Only controlled, prospective, therapeutic trials can settle this question, and the evidence to date, while admittedly incomplete, is not encouraging.

EVIDENCE FROM THERAPEUTIC TRIALS

The Veterans Administration study

The most comprehensive controlled trial is the US Veterans Administration study[13–15]. This study included 520 male patients with initial diastolic blood pressure in the range 90–129 mmHg. The patients were at higher risk than those generally encountered in practice. They exhibited more evidence of target organ disease and about 20% had previous major complications. Furthermore, one of the criteria for inclusion was that the patient must remain hypertensive during a period of hospitalization. Patients were also selected on the basis of good compliance, for the obvious reason that the trial was designed to test the effectiveness of treatment, *per se*, on morbidity and mortality. The patients were randomly assigned double-blind either to the triple-drug regimen of hydrochlorothiazide plus reserpine plus hydralazine or to placebos of these agents.

Overall results
Because of conclusive evidence of benefit in the severe group the trial was discontinued early in the 143 patients with diastolic levels of 115–129 mmHg. This group exhibited hypertensive complications almost exclusively, and these were prevented in activity treated patients. However, in the 380 patients with initial diastolic levels of 90–114 mmHg the trial was continued longer with an average follow-up of 3·3 years and in some cases over 5 years. Nineteen cardiovascular-related deaths occurred in the control group versus only eight in the treated patients. Death due to haemorrhagic stroke and dissecting aortic aneurysm occurred only in the control patients, whereas myocardial infarction, sudden death and atherothrombotic stroke occurred in both groups.

All major morbid events, whether fatal or nonfatal, were analysed by the life-table method of analysis. This analysis, which was projected over a 5-year period of follow-up, indicated an incidence of major complications occurring in 56% of the control group versus 18% of the treated patients. The difference in morbidity, therefore, was three to one in favour of treatment.

Differing results in mild versus moderate hypertension
When mild and moderate hypertensive patients were analysed separately the difference in the incidence of major complications was four to one in favour of treatment in the moderate group, but was less than two to one in the mild group and in the latter did not reach the

level of statistical significance. In searching for the reason for an apparent lack of significant benefit in the mild group it was noted that the complications in that group were almost exclusively of the atherosclerotic type, principally myocardial infarction, heart-blocks and atrial fibrillation.

Further analysis of the data as to type of complication indicated that the treated patients exhibited complete protection against congestive heart failure, renal failure, dissecting aortic aneurysm and accelerated hypertension. A total of 10% of the control patients versus none of the treated cases exhibited progression of their hypertension to diastolic levels of 125 mmHg or higher, requiring removal from the trial and substitution of active treatment. Strokes occurred in only one-fourth as many patients in the treated group as in the control group of patients. It was only with respect to the various complications of coronary artery disease that the treated and non-treated patients exhibited a similar incidence. This again emphasizes the lack of effectiveness of treatment on atherosclerotic complications as opposed to hypertensive complications, and explains why the patients with mild hypertension who develop atherosclerotic complications predominantly did not achieve greater benefit.

The US Public Health Service Hospitals study
Another major controlled trial has been carried out by Smith and his associates in the US Public Health Service Hospitals. The results have, thus far, been published only in abstract form[16]. This study included 389 male and female patients who were followed up for 7 years. Unlike the Veterans Administration study this trial excluded patients with evidence of target organ disease. Although both mild and moderate grades of severity of hypertension were included the patients were predominantly mild and also rather young, the average age being 44 years.

Differing effectiveness against atherosclerotic and hypertensive complications
The results of the Public Health Service trial confirmed in general those of the Veterans Administration study. Treatment provided significant protection against hypertensive complicatons but not against atherosclerotic complications of the coronary arteries including myocardial infarction. It should be noted that the patients in this trial were on the average younger and had less advanced disease than the population in the Veterans Administration study. Also, the period of follow-up was longer, an important consideration in dealing with such a slowly progressive disorder as atherosclerosis. Despite these more favourable circumstances, however, there still was no evidence that normalization of blood pressure prevented the regression of coronary artery disease and appearance of its

complications.

Why does treatment fail to prevent atherosclerotic complications?
The apparent failure of antihypertensive therapy to prevent atherosclerotic complications appears at first glance to be paradoxical. As already indicated hypertension aggravates and accelerates atherosclerosis[12]. Why then shouldn't reduction of an elevated blood pressure arrest the progress of the vascular lesion, as appears to be the case with hypertensive complications? What is different about atherosclerosis? In the absence of definitive evidence the most likely hypothesis is that hypertension produces, in the arterial wall, irreversible changes that predispose to the development of atherosclerosis regardless of the subsequent level of the blood pressure. Recent evidence indicates that atherosclerosis begins as a result of injury to the arterial intima[17]. Smooth muscle cells in the arterial wall migrate into the area of injury where they proliferate. This is followed by connective tissue hyperplasia and lipid deposition resulting in atherosclerosis. Hypertension produces marked alterations in the arterial wall including fragmentation of elastic tissue lamellae, proliferation of connective tissue and deposition of collagen. Such changes make the wall less compliant and possibly more subject to injury in addition to the stress of the elevated pressure, *per se*. It is noteworthy that these changes in the arterial wall are similar to those found in aged normotensive persons who are also prone to develop atherosclerosis. It is a reasonable speculation that the arteries of both younger hypertensive and older normotensives are responding to the same process of 'wear and tear' but that the process is accelerated in hypertensives because of the higher level of blood pressure. The vascular injuries initiating the atherosclerotic process are produced at a relatively early stage of the hypertension and the lesions once formed apparently are not reversed by lowering the blood pressure. (An interesting consequence of this hypothesis is that for effective prevention of atherosclerosis treatment of the entire population should be undertaken from an early age so as to maintain the lowest possible level of blood pressure within the limits of comfort. However, the evidence available at present obviously does not justify such a drastic approach.)

INDICATIONS FOR TREATMENT

Indications for moderate and severe essential hypertension
The most important conclusion to be drawn from the presently available evidence is as follows: antihypertensive drug treatment is indicated whenever, in the judgment of the physician, the risk of developing

hypertensive complications is high. This means that all patients with a diastolic blood pressure averaging 105 mmHg or higher (fifth phase) over three or more clinic or office visits should receive treatment. Again, it is necessary to emphasize that the patient cannot be classified as to severity on the basis of one or even two visits, as the initial visit may be quite misleading.

Indications for mild hypertension
The treatment of patients with diastolic levels averaging in the mild range 90–104 mmHg is not so well defined. Treatment may be indicated in some but not in others. The selection of patients in the mild range for treatment is based on various criteria which reflect increased risk of morbidity and mortality. These criteria are as follows:

Age
For any given level of blood pressure the younger the patient the greater is the reduction in life expectancy. Life insurance statistics show that for a blood pressure of 150/100 mmHg the 20-year mortality for men in the age range of 50–59 is twice normal, whereas in the age range 30–39 it is five times normal[8].

Sex
Women appear to tolerate hypertension better than men. Various studies indicate that mortality rates are approximately 1·5–2·0 times higher in men than in women[6,18].

Race
Although it may not be possible to generalize worldwide, the black residents of the United States show a considerably greater mortality from hypertension as compared with whites. The death-rate for hypertensive black men was four times higher than in white men[19]. The excess mortality is particularly high in black patients below the age of 50, who seem prone to develop severe or accelerated hypertension.

Lability of blood pressure
It is not generally appreciated how much blood pressure will fluctuate over a 24 h period. Using a portable recorder[20] the blood pressure in a normal subject was shown to fluctuate between 75/40 mmHg (during sleep) and 140/90 mmHg over a 24 h period with brief peaks to 150/90 mmHg once during a painful stimulus and again during coitus. In a hypertensive patient the fluctuation was from 160/65 to 270/170 mmHg. The lowest values always occur during sleep and the highest levels during a strong emotional stimulus. Since a visit to a

doctor's office is often associated with some apprehension it is apparent that readings obtained there will usually be near the high extreme of the diurnal variation.

Some hypertensive patients exhibit greater fluctuation of blood pressure than others. Those exhibiting the greatest fluctuation with frequent drops into the normotensive range may be described as having labile hypertension. These individuals have a considerably better prognosis and exhibit less target organ disease than the patients who are less labile[21,22]. Lability of hypertension is best determined by having the blood pressure recorded in the home twice daily for a period of several weeks. A member of the patient's family can be taught by the office nurse to take the blood pressure. This is an especially helpful procedure in patients who exhibit persistently high office readings without any evidence of target organ disease.

Family history
Essential hypertension has a strong genetic component[23]. In identical twins if hypertension occurs in one member of the pair it will also occur in the other. Even the severity of the hypertension appears to be similar in both twins[24]. A history of relatively early death in a parent or sibling from a complication such as stroke, renal failure or congestive heart failure increases the likelihood of progression in the patient with mild hypertension.

Target organ disease
Evidence of damage to the major target organs, heart, brain and kidney, is perhaps the most important index of severity second only to the average level of blood pressure[6,14,25]. In the Veterans Administration cooperative study the incidence of cardiovascular complications in untreated patients with average diastolic blood pressure in the range 90–115 mmHg was two and one-half times higher in the patients exhibiting target organ disease at the time of entry than in those who had no signs of organic damage[15].

Hyperlipidaemia and diabetes mellitus
Unlike the prognostic indices described above hyperlipidaemia and diabetes are not related to progression of hypertension, *per se*, but rather they indicate increased risk of developing atherosclerosis of the coronary arteries. The most important known risk factors for coronary artery disease are hypercholesterolaemia and elevated blood pressure. Less important but still significant prognostic indices are cigarette-smoking, diabetes mellitus, obesity and lack of physical exercise[26]. These various indices are additive, so that patients who have a combination of risk factors have

a considerably worsened prognosis than those who do not. Therefore, the hypertensive patient who has an elevated serum cholesterol or blood sugar or other risk factors is at relatively high risk of developing coronary artery disease.

The implications of these epidemiological observations with respect to treatment is not clear. No matter how rational the reduction of serum cholesterol or blood sugar level may seem it has not yet been shown that such treatment results in effective prevention of coronary artery disease. However, the opposite is also true, since it has not been proven that reduction of risk factors by dietary therapeutic or hygienic measures is of *no* value. Unfortunately, definitive data on which to base a sound judgment are lacking at this time.

The failure to prevent atherosclerotic complications by controlling hypertension has already been alluded to. Although hypercholesterolaemia and diabetes mellitus may be of value in indicating increased risk of atherosclerotic complications they are not predictors of *hypertensive* complications. Since treatment has been shown to prevent the latter but not the former, the presence of hypercholesterolaemia and diabetes have only questionable significance in predicting any benefit to be derived from antihypertensive treatment. Hopefully, this conclusion will in the future be reversed by intervention trials at present taking place on the control of mild hypertension and other risk factors.

Guidelines for treatment
The following guidelines for instituting antihypertensive treatment utilize existing knowledge presently available from controlled therapeutic trials. The rationale on which the guidelines are formulated is based on the principle that antihypertensive therapy is indicated whenever there is an increased risk of hypertensive complications. If at some future time evidence is obtained for prevention of atherosclerotic complications then the indications for treatment should be broadened to include all patients with blood pressure of 140/90 mmHg or above.

For patients with diastolic levels averaging 105 mmHg or above
All patients, whether male or female, old or young, of any race should receive treatment if the diastolic blood pressure during *three or more* separate office or clinic visits averages 105 mmHg or more. Whereas the Veterans Administration study was limited to males with persistent hypertension and considerable end-organ damage the US Public Health Service trial included patients of both sexes and no detectable end-organ disease[16]. Prospective epidemiological studies also indicate that all patients with diastolic levels of 105 mmHg or above are at risk of developing hypertensive, as well as atherosclerotic, complications.

For patients with diastolic levels averaging 90–104 mmHg
No hard and fast rules can be made for the management of patients with diastolic blood pressure averaging below 105 mmHg. The physician has the option of following these patients without treatment, or he may choose to treat selected individuals in this group. In making the decision for treatment the physician should consider the other indices of risk enumerated above as well as the level of blood pressure. For example, a black male age 35 with a diastolic blood pressure averaging 95 mmHg should be treated, whereas a 60-year-old female with a similar level of average diastolic blood pressure probably should not.

Risk factors rating scale   In an attempt to formalize therapeutic indications in patients with average diastolic levels in the range of 90–104 mmHg this author has utilized a rating scale in which a score of one point is given for the presence of each of the following risk factors:

> male
> black
> under 45 years old
> either parent with major hypertensive complications
> diastolic above 95 at all of three office visits.

A score of 2 is given for the presence of target organ involvement (Group II fundi changes, left ventricular hypertrophy, proteinurea, etc.). The scores are added together to obtain the summed risk index. The criteria for treatment are then as follows:

Diastolic Average	Summed Risk Index
90–94	4 or more
95–99	3 or more
100–104	2 or more

These guidelines provide an objective method for selecting patients with mild hypertension who are most likely to benefit from antihypertensive therapy. They can be varied somewhat according to individual circumstance. Patients with mild hypertension who are not treated must be checked at approximately yearly intervals since at least 10% will progress to a more severe stage.

CONCLUSIONS

Antihypertensive drug treatment is effective in preventing many of the major complications associated with hypertension. The preventable com-

plications include stroke, particularly cerebral and subarachnoid haemorrhage; congestive heart failure; malignant hypertension; renal failure;
dissecting aortic aneurysm and progression of the hypertension to a more
severe stage. More widespread recognition of this advance by the profession and the public should be followed by a significant fall in
death-rate associated with *moderate* and *severe* hypertension.

In patients with mild hypertension myocardial infarction and 'sudden
death' are by far the major causes of death. At present, evidence is lacking that antihypertensive treatment protects against these atherosclerotic complications. Nevertheless, treatment is effective against some
complications that may occur in mild hypertension, such as the electrocardiographic manifestations of left ventricular hypertrophy and it prevents progression of the hypertension to a more severe stage. Although
the available evidence may not justify the mass treatment of mild
patients it should be followed (since they may progress) and some who
are at higher risk than others probably should be treated.

References

1 Hatano, S. (1975). Hypertension in Japan: A review. In O. Paul (ed.). *Epidemiology and Control of Hypertension*, pp. 63–99. (New York and London: Stratton
Intercontinental Medical Book Corporation)

2 Aleksandrow, D. (1967). Studies on the epidemiology of hypertension in Poland. In
J. Stamler, R. Stamler and T. N. Pullman (eds.). *The Epidemiology of Hypertension*, pp. 82–97. (New York and London: Grune and Stratton)

3 Shaper, A. G. (1972). Cardiovascular disease in the tropics. III. Blood pressure and
hypertension. *Br. Med. J.*, **3**, 805

4 National Center for Health Statistics (1964). Blood pressure of adults by race and
area, United States 1960–1962. *Vital and Health Statistics*. PHS Pub. No. 1000,
Series 11. No. 5

5 Freis, E. D. (1976). Salt, volume and the prevention of hypertension. *Circulation*,
53, 473

6 Sokolow, M. and Perloff, D. (1961). The prognosis of essential hypertension
treated conservatively. *Circulation*, **23**, 697

7 Kannel, W. B. (1969). Some factors affecting morbidity and mortality in hypertension. *Milbank Mem. Fund. Q.*, **74**, 116

8 *Society of Actuaries Data on Build and Blood Pressure Study* (1959). Vol. I. (Chicago: Society of Actuaries)

9 National Health Survey: Hypertension and hypertensive heart disease in adults.
United States 1960–1962. Washington, DC, US Department of Health, Education
and Welfare. *Vital and Health Statistics*, Series 11, No. 13, US Government Print-
ing Office, 1966

10 Carey, R. M., Reid, R.A., Ayers, C. R., Lyrich, S. S., McLain, W. L. and
Vaugh, E. D., Jr. (1976). The Charlottesville blood-pressure survey. Value of repeated blood pressure measurements. *J. Am. Med. Assoc.*, **236**, 847

11 Heyden, S., Bortel, A. G., Hamer, C. G. and McDonough, J. R. (1969). Elevated
blood pressure levels in adolescents, Evans County, Georgia. *J. Am. Med. Assoc.*,
209, 1683

12 Fries, E. D. (1969). Hypertension and atherosclerosis. *Am. J. Med.*, **46,** 735
13 Veterans Administration Cooperative Study Group on Antihypertensive Agents (1967). Effects of treatment in morbidity in hypertension. Results in patients with diastolic blood pressures averaging 115 through 129 mmHg. *J. Am. Med. Assoc.*, **202,** 1028
14 Veterans Administration Cooperative Study Group on Antihypertensive Agents (1970). II. Results in patients with diastolic blood pressure averaging 90 through 114 mmHg. *J. Am. Med. Assoc.*, **213,** 1143
15 Veterans Administration Cooperative Study Group on Antihypertensive Agents (1972). III. Influence of age, diastolic blood pressure, prior cardio-vascular disease. Further analysis of side effects. *Circulation*, **45,** 991
16 Smith, W. McF. (1976). Intervention trial in mild hypertension. Cooperative Study Group, Public Health Service Hospitals. *Circulation*, 95 (Suppl. II) 95
17 Ross, R. and Glomset, J. A. (1976). The pathogenesis of artherosclerosis. *N. Engl. J. Med.*, **295,** 369
18 Bechgaard, P. (1946). Arterial hypertension; follow-up study of one thousand hypertonics. *Acta Med. Scand.* (Suppl., 1972), 3
19 Vital Statistics of the United States, 1967. Section 6, Mortality Statistics, US Depaartment of Health, Education and Welfare. Public Health Service, National Center for Health
20 Pickering, G. (1968). *High Blood Pressure.* Ed. 2, 717, pp. 53–57 (New York: Grune and Stratton)
21 Smirk, F. H., Veal, A M. D. and Olstad, K. S. (1959). Basal and supplemental blood pressure in relation to life expectancy and hypertension symptomatology. *NZ Med. J.*, **53,** 711
22 Mathisen, H. S., Jensen, D., Loken, E. and Loken, H. (1959). The prognosis in essential hypertension. *Am. Heart J.*, **57,** 371
23 Schweitzer, M. D., Chark, E. G., Gearing, F. R. and Perera, G. A. (1962). Genetic factors in primary hypertension and coronary disease. *J. Chron. Dis.*, **45,** 1093
24 Platt, R. (1963). Heredity in hypertension. *Lancet*, **i,** 899
25 Palmer, R. S. and Muench, H. (1953). Course and prognosis of essential hypertension. Follow-up of 453 patients ten years after original series was closed. *J. Am. Med. Assoc.*, **153,** 1
26 Truett, J., Cornfield, J. and Kannel, W.B. (1967). A multivariate analysis of the risk of coronary heart disease in Framingham. *J. Chronic Dis.*, **20,** 511

2

Screening and community control of hypertension

R. Reader

INTRODUCTION

An organized public health programme for the control of hypertensive disease now offers one of the most rewarding opportunities of our time, presenting a notable challenge to both traditional medical practice and to public health services. It must involve screening procedures to identify symptomless hypertension and active measures to bring those found to be hypertensive under effective management.

There is no need to elaborate here on the extent of the medical and socioeconomic consequences of raised blood pressure in the community, though it should be emphasized that life insurance data[1], the Framingham Study[2,3], and the Pooling Project[4] have shown that these consequences are not confined to the severe levels of hypertension. Morbidity and mortality from hypertensive diseases increase significantly as pressures rise, even through what are commonly regarded as normal levels.

Screening for symptomless hypertension is not new. It has long been standard practice to exclude individuals from life insurance, the armed services or employment by various institutions, particularly government. If hypertension was diagnosed the individual was excluded and the object of the procedure achieved. The procedure had nothing to do with the welfare of the individual; in fact, quite the contrary. It is true that in recent years many such patients, particularly those with severe degrees of hypertension, did benefit in that they consulted their doctor and went on to effective therapy, but this was incidental to the objective.

But all of this is no longer true; the opportunity is now available to approach screening for hypertension with the positive objective of reducing morbidity and mortality in the community. The reversal in the role of screening has come about as the result of three advances: the appreciation of the high prevalence of symptomless hypertension in the community, the availability of effective hypotensive drugs and the demonstration of the benefits of therapy in the large number in the community with symptomless and moderate levels of hypertension.

THE HIGH PREVALENCE OF HYPERTENSION

It has been known for many years that hypertension is a common disease. Janeway[5] in 1913 reported systolic blood pressures above 160 mmHg in 11% of 7872 subjects and May[6], in 1925, reported levels above 140 mmHg in 25% of men and 17.4% of women life-insurance candidates. There have been many other similar reports of high prevalence, but they caused little reaction. The studies were usually in selected populations and their validity uncertain. In any case, accurate estimates of prevalence of disease in a community only matter if resources have to be devoted to its control, and, until recently, there was no question of an organized programme to deal with hypertension.

USA national survey on hypertension
It was fortuitious that, just as other indications were falling into place that hypertension was a public health problem susceptible to public health measures, the United States Public Health Service[7] in 1966 published the results of its very significant survey of prevalence of hypertension in the American community. The 7710 subjects, identified by the sample design as representative of the entire community, were invited by door-to-door canvass to participate, and 6672 (82%) were examined by physicians based in mobile units using methods which had been pretested and demonstrated to give reproducible and reliable results. The blood pressure was taken as the average of three readings recorded seated, at intervals throughout the 2 h examination. Definite hypertension was taken as 160 mmHg or more systolic, and 95 mmHg or more diastolic, phase 5. Among adults, 15.3% of those aged 18–79 years were hypertensive by these criteria. This figure has been confirmed by other surveys in many countries[8–11] (see Table 1).

Effect of age, sex, race and occupation on prevalence
Figures 1 and 2 (reproduced from the Report of 1966[7]) illustrate the increasing prevalence with age of both hypertension and hypertensive heart disease, the higher prevalence in white males under 50 and the crossover to higher prevalence in females over that age, and the very high prevalence in negroes of both sexes and at all ages. There were variations

Table 1 Prevalence of hypertension (DBP $\geqslant$ 95 mmHg) in both sexes in certain age groups in four countries

Author	Date of survey	Number examined	Prevalence (%)				Population	BP measurement	Observer
			15–29	30–44	45–50	60+			
USPHS[7] (USA)	1960–62	6672	1·6	9·3	19·8	34·9	Sample of whole population re-cruited by house-hold visit	Average of three readings, single visit seated, Phase V	Physicians
Wilber[11] (USA)	1962	3084	3·0	11·4	22·3	24·4	Community sample by household visit 45% non-white	Average of three readings at single visit seated	Nurses
Hamilton et al., [9] (UK)	1954	2031	2·6	6·4	18·7	38·3	Hospital out-patient, non-medical patients	Single reading seated, Phase IV	Physicians
Boe et al.[8] (Norway)	1950–51	36 093	3·3	9·0	22·4	35·9	Whole community at X-ray attend-ance	Seated, lowest reading, single measurement, Phase IV	Nurses
McCall et al.[10] (Australia)	1966	3392	3·7	7·9	16·6	19·7	Whole community at health survey	Seated, lowest reading, single measurement, Phase IV	Physicians

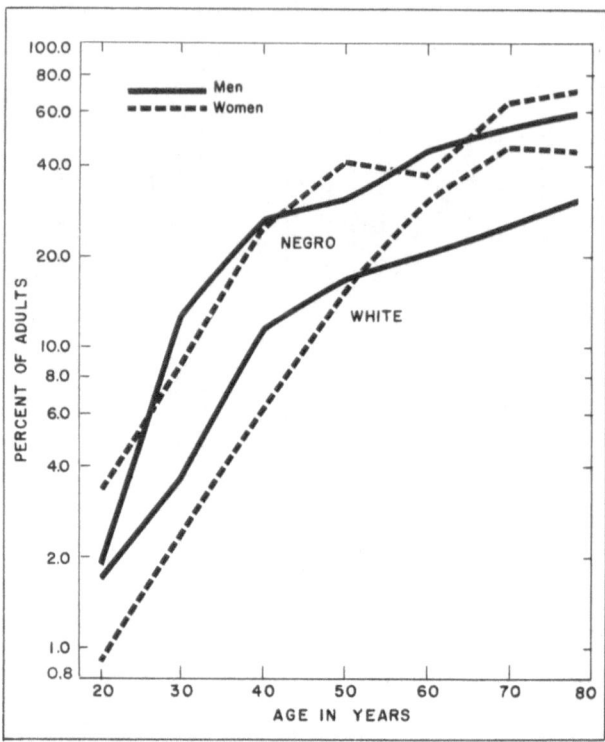

Figure 1 Percentage of adults with definite hypertension, by age, race and sex. From Ref. 7

in prevalence by geographic region throughout the USA, being generally high in the north-east and low in the west; high in rural and low in urban non-metropolitan areas. Prevalence was higher in lower income groups and with lower levels of education both for men and women and for whites and non-whites. Professional workers had a low prevalence, and service workers and farm labourers a high prevalence, both in white and non-white males. The prevalence of hypertensive heart disease paralleled hypertension in all these sub-sets.

Notwithstanding the previous reports of high prevalence of hypertension, the results of this survey were arresting and put the problem of hypertension in an entirely new light.

DEVELOPMENT OF DRUG THERAPY

The advent of hypotensive drugs
It was 130 years after Bright's first recognition of hypertension as a clini-

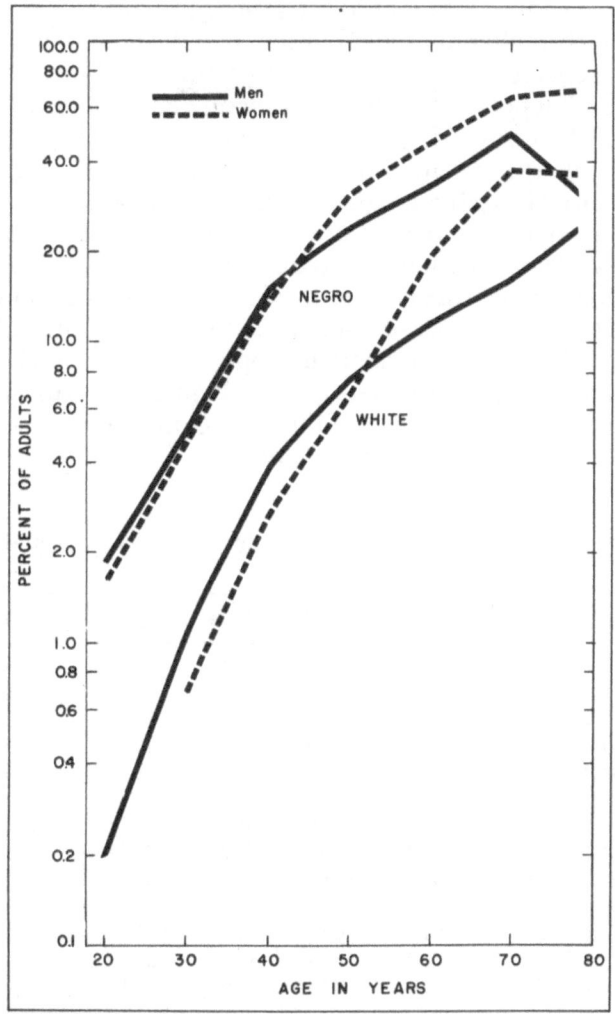

Figure 2 Percentage of adults with hypertensive heart disease, by age, race and sex. From Ref. 7

cal problem (in the 1820s), before a clearly effective form of therapy emerged. Apart from those rare cases in which a primary cause could be dealt with surgically, treatment remained non-specific, symptomatic and largely ineffective throughout this period. An uneasy exception in the 1940s was the brief era of lumbodorsal sympathectomy. The undertaking of this heroic surgery with intangible benefits (the headaches appeared to be relieved even if the blood pressure was little changed)

The Treatment of Hypertension

testified to the wide acceptance of the serious prognosis of hypertension, and particularly malignant hypertension, and the length to which physicians were prepared to go in an effort to control it. The procedure was dropped like a hot potato and the whole picture changed in 1950 with the introduction of pharmacological agents which reduced blood pressure by modifying sympathetic control of the circulation.

The sequential introduction of new and effective agents since then has been an impressive achievement of the pharmaceutical industry. Pentamethonium and hexamethonium products were first used in Australia in 1950; pentolinium tartrate became available in 1953, the rauwolfia products in the same year, mecamylamine in 1957, chlorothiazide in 1958, guanethidine in 1960, alphamethyldopa in 1962, and the beta-adrenergic antagonists were first used for high blood pressure in 1970. The trend in usage and the costs of these drugs in Australia over the past few years are shown in Table 2 and Figure 3.

Table 2   **Drugs for hypertension – prescription costs in $000 – Australia***
(1972–76)

	1972	*1973*	*1974*	*1975*	*1976*
Methyldopa	7977	8649	9112	9778	11 987
Clonidine			974	1681	2127
Guanethedine	2373	2220	2033	1850	1752
Debrisequine	806	1056	1132	1200	1484
Rauwolfia	1078	1061	1312	1057	596
Frusemide	4581	5138	5567	6237	7622
Chlorothiazide	2470	2737	3224	3759	4896
Chlorthalidone	1510	1934	2001	2050	2312
Propranolol	477	660	1226	1173	4895
Prindolol	10	339	1237	2400	3843
Oxprenolol	159	224	264	449	1277

* By courtesy Australian Department of Health.

The value of these drugs in severe symptomatic and malignant hypertension was immediately apparent in clinical practice, and these clinical impressions were quickly substantiated by a number of small therapeutic trials summarized in Table 3[12–16]. Their use, however, continued in the traditional doctor–patient therapeutic system. Treatment was instituted when the patient sought medical aid for the relief of symptoms, or occasionally if severe hypertension was discovered in other ways.

While individual patient management was thus revolutionized, for the

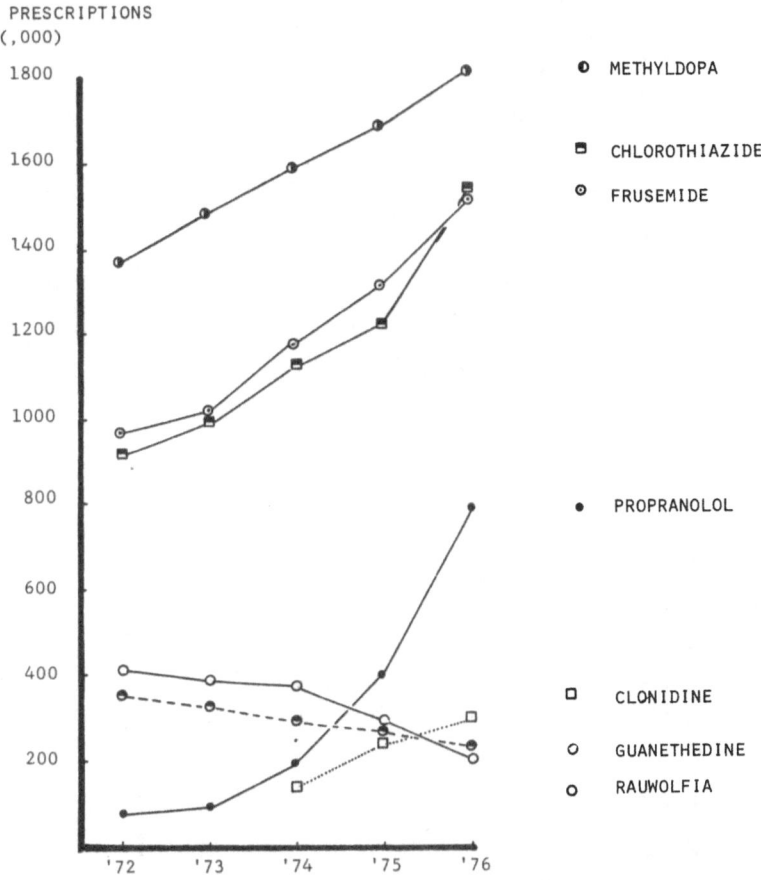

Figure 3   Trends in numbers of prescriptions for hypotensive drugs in Australia,
1972–76

first 15 years of pharmacological therapy for hypertension, there was
little thought given to the possibility that the drugs were contributing at
a broad community level, or that they could form the basis of a public
health programme. Trees were falling, but few noticed the effect on the
woods. But falling mortality from hypertensive heart disease and cerebrovascular disease in adults under 65 occurred in a number of countries in the 1950s and 1960s (Table 4)[17]. The age-adjusted trend for
mortality from cerebrovascular disease under age 65 in Australia is il-
lustrated in Figure 4[18]. The premise that this fall was due to pharmacological treatment of hypertension has been discussed with reservations
by Moriyama *et al.*[17], and Paul[19], who point out that mortality rates

Table 3 Therapeutic trials in severe hypertension

	Number of patients		Type of patients	Period	Type of endpoint	Endpoints	
	Treated	Control				Treated	Control
Leishman [12]	183	104	Male and female	5 years	Mortality, stroke, uraemia	Death-rate reduced to one-third	
Hamilton [13]	30	31	Male and female	2–6 years	Strokes	3	7
Marshall [14]	39	42	Male and female Treated mean 42 years Controls mean 60 years Recovered from stroke or	3 years	Death. Non-Fatal CVA	4 8	12 22
Wolff and Lindeman [15]	45	42	Mainly non-white; mean	2 years		6	19
Veterans Administrative Cooperative Study [16]	73	70	Males, 30–73	4 months– 2 years	Death. severe hypertensive complication	0 2	4 27

DBP = diastolic blood pressure; CVA = Cerebrovascular accident

Table 4 Death-rates for cerebrovascular diseases per 100 000 population, age 55–64, by sex: sixteen countries, 1950 and 1960 (ICD code B22)

	Male			Female		
Country	1950	1960	Percentage change	1950	1960	Percentage change
South Africa (white)	200·0	223·7	+ 11·9	215·0	221·1	+ 2·8
Canada	165·9	135·4	− 18·4	177·9	115·8	− 34·9
United States (white)	182·2	139·0	− 23·7	156·9	103·0	− 34·4
Japan	437·3	610·9	+ 39·7	367·9	367·1	− 0·2
Austria*	215·2	207·8	− 3·4	163·8	135·5	− 18·8
Belgium†	72·7	92·2	+ 26·8	60·3	62·3	+ 3·3
Denmark‡	139·3	106·5	− 23·5	154·6	84·9	− 45·1
England and Wales	194·5	187·8	− 3·4	187·3	155·2	− 17·1
Italy‡	229·7	207·0	− 9·9	186·3	148·5	− 20·3
Norway‡	114·9	117·3	+ 2·1	134·2	119·6	− 10·9
Netherlands	102·2	94·6	− 7·4	126·4	85·4	− 32·4
Scotland	237·3	241·6	+ 1·8	255·5	198·5	− 22·3
Sweden‡	161·4	131·9	− 18·3	185·2	110·7	− 40·2
Switzerland‡	176·7	119·9	− 32·1	170·1	93·7	− 44·9
Australia	235·1	201·1	− 14·5	233·7	172·4	− 26·2
New Zealand	132·8	152·0	+ 14·5	192·9	147·6	− 23·5

Source: Numbers of deaths are from World Health Organization, Annual Epidemiological and Vital Statistics. Populations are from United Nations Demographic Yearbook, 1962.
* Rate in 1950 column is for 1953.
† Rate in 1950 column is for 1954.
‡ Rate in 1950 column is for 1951.
Data reproduced from Ref. 17.

for hypertensive diseases were falling before 1950 in the USA and that it was unlikely that the number of patients in whom medical treatment was applied effectively was large enough to account for substantial savings in lives. However, analysis of the Australian experience in terms of the actual numbers of deaths from cerebrovascular disease in relation to the numbers of patients on effective hypotensive therapy[18], presented in Table 5, is consistent with the conclusion that pharmacological therapy was influencing national mortality statistics. The data on numbers of hypertensives and numbers on treatment are based on three epidemiological studies[10,20,21]. The matter is discussed more fully elsewhere[18].

The scale of benefit: therapeutic trials
The scale of benefit of treatment in severe hypertension was demon-

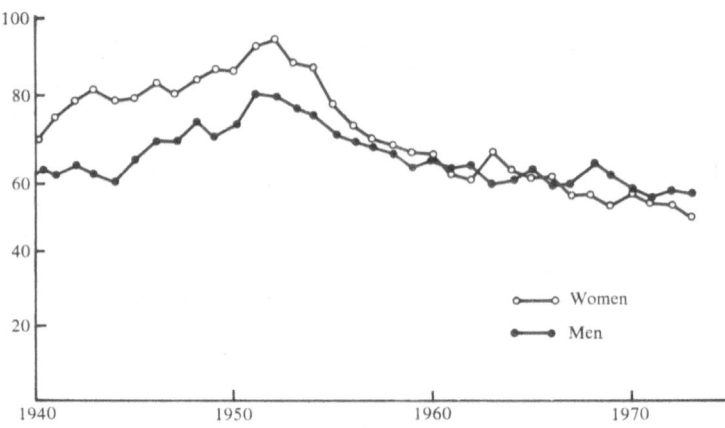

Figure 4   Age-adjusted mortality rates per 100 000 for cerebrovascular disease in Australia for men and women aged 30–64 years, 1940–73. From Ref. 18

strated in the early 1960s in a series of small therapeutic trials previously referred to (Table 3). Follow-up periods varied from 2 to 6 years, the patients were suffering from severe or symptomatic hypertension, and morbidity and mortality were one-third or less in the treated group compared with the controls. The results were consistent with clinical experience, and predictable. But in the 1960s it was standard practice not to treat hypertension of mild degree and, indeed, to avoid even advising the patients of its existence.

Table 5   Estimation of effect of treatment on mortality from CVA, Australia 1973

	Number	Expected deaths* Not treated	Treated	Lives saved by treatment	Calculated lives saved from fall in mortality 1951–73
Population (age 30–64)	7 547 222				
Hypertensives	1 230 100	13 352			
Hypertensives on treatment	550 945				
Hypertensives on effective treatment	188 680	2075	320	1745	1872

Data reproduced from Ref. 18.

Expected deaths calculated from Veterans Administration Study, 1967–70.

The critical study which dramatically changed attitudes to milder forms of hypertension, and particularly symptomless hypertension, was that of the Veterans Administration Cooperative Group which commenced in 1965 and reported its results in 1967[16] and 1970[22]. The first phase confirmed earlier studies that severe hypertension (diastolic greater than 114 mmHg) was dramatically improved with hypotensive therapy (see Table 3). The results in the 186 treated and 194 control male patients with mild and moderate hypertension (diastolic 90–114 mmHg) were reported in 1970. Mean age was 51 years and duration of study 1 to 5.5 years. There were 8 deaths from cardiovascular causes in treated, compared to 19 in control, subjects and terminating events other than death occurred in only 1 treated compared with 16 controls.

The significance of this study in mild and moderate hypertension was to indicate benefit in a much larger proportion of the hypertensive population than had previously been envisaged. The results dramatically drew the attention of medical authorities throughout the entire world to the potential benefit of an organized programme to prevent hypertensive complications in the community. Although the study, of necessity, left many vital questions unanswered, it undoubtedly launched a worldwide activity in screening for, and treatment of, symptomless hypertension.

Subsequent analyses of the results[23] indicated that, in the hypertensive population studied, the benefit from therapy was largely concentrated in those with diastolic pressures above 105 mmHg, in the older age groups and in those with already manifest target organ damage.

One of the great merits of the study was also one of its limitations. To define precisely the blood pressure of each subject a careful preparatory phase was conducted, including several days' rest in hospital, during which those with variable and labile pressures, and also non-compliant patients were identified and excluded. The study was confined to men. These measures, while ensuring a homogeneous study population, have proved difficult as regards translating the results to screening procedures involving assessment of casual blood pressures, that are feasible in a widespread community approach to the detection of symptomless hypertension. They also leave undetermined the scale of benefits that will occur in women, in subjects with labile hypertension and in the open community where the benefits of drug therapy will be diluted in a less compliant population.

There are now other therapeutic trials in progress in various parts of the world designed to investigate further the relationships between mild hypertension and drug therapy[24] (see Tables 6, 7, and 8). It may be some years before the results of these are available, but in the meantime the Veterans Administration Study provided the third and vital compon-

Table 6 Some features of eight therapeutic trials in mild hypertension

Study	Age (years)	Sex	Commenced	Comments
Cooperative study of hypertension, USA (USPHS)	⩽55	M and F	Sept. 1966	Multi-centric in 6 USPHS hospitals. Study in mariners, hospital employees, coastguards, etc.
Hypertension detection and follow-up programme, NHLBI, USA (HDFP)	30–69	M and F	Feb. 1973	Fourteen centres, recruitment by house-to-house screening. Subjects randomised step care v. regular care
Cooperative study, USA (VA–NIH)	21–49	M and F	Jan. 1974	Multi-centric based on VA hospitals. Subjects recruited from veterans, their families and others associated with the hospital. In feasibility stage
Treatment trial for mild hypertension, UK (MRC)	35–64	M and F	Mar. 1973	Multi-centric trial. Subjects recruited from general practice or industrial groups or hospital clinics. Feasibility stage complete. Scientific and ethical feasibility demonstrated
St Thomas's Hospital, UK	35–64	M	Jun. 1972	Feasibility study. In patients of a group general practice
National blood pressure study, Australia (NBPS)	30–69	M and F	Jul. 1973	Screening conducted in general population in four centres
European working party in hypertension the elderly, (EWPHE)	>60	M and F	Jan. 1973	Fifteen centres. One-year pilot study in 140 patients completed
Groupe d'Études sur L'épidémiologie de L'athérosclerose, Paris (GREA)	⩽59	M and F	Oct. 1972	In personnel of Paris police force

Data reproduced from Ref. 25.

Table 7   Some features of eight therapeutic trials in mild hypertension, criteria and methodology – blood pressure measurement, therapeutic trials in hypertension

Study	DBP-range	Sphygmo-manometer	No. of readings per visit	No. of visits	Computation of definitive pressure
USPHS	90–114	Standard	2	3	Mean of 4*
HDFP	>90	RZ	2	3	Mean of 4
VA–NIH	85–104	Automatic	3	3	Mean of 9
MRC	90–109	RZ	2	2	Mean of 4
St Thomas's	90–114	RZ	2	2	Mean of 4
NBPS	95–109	RZ	2	2	Mean of 4
EWPHE	90–119	Standard	1†	3	Mean of 3‡
GREA	95–115	Standard	2	2	Mean of 4

* After 3 months run-in on placebo.
† After 1 month run-in on placebo.
‡ The third of three readings.
RZ = random zero.
Data reproduced from Ref. 25.

ent establishing the case for a public health programme for control of hypertension and its complications.

The case established
It was clear by 1970 that hypertension could be effectively controlled by drug therapy, that it was of such widespread prevalence as to be a major public health problem, and finally that serious disability and death could be prevented in the significant number in the community with symptomless and relatively mild hypertension.

COMPONENTS OF A CONTROL PROGRAMME

In the course of the therapeutic trials referreto above, and as a result of experience in community control programmes already undertaken[26–28], many of the problems associated with the techniques and methods of such community programmes have been defined. These concern the technique of measuring blood pressure, methods of identifying all hypertensives in the community, the role of specialized investigations for primary cause, the logistics of medical management of the hypertensives identified, time of starting drug therapy, the choice of drugs and the management of drug therapy, the maintenance of patient cooperation and compliance in the long-term management, and a back-up community and professional education programme.

Table 8 Some features of eight therapeutic trials in mild hypertension. Trial population – numbers by age – men and women

	<30	30-34	35-39	40-44	45-49	50-54	55-59	60-64	65-69	>69	All ages	Total feasibility	Planned full study
USPHS	13	20	51	84	143	67	11				389		389
HDFP		716	962	1363	1787	2008	1685	1345	976		10 842		10 842
VA–NIH*	176	151	168	217	225						937	1600	8000
MRC*	9	24	126	236	390	443	310	196			1734	2000	18 000
St Thomas's			5	20	22	18	16	20			101		101
NBPS		227	334	482	780	837	666	431	198		3955		3955
EWPHE*									43	102	145		1000
GREA*	3	2	10	41	34	43	5				138		2000
TOTALS	201	1140	1656	2443	3381	3416	2693	1992	1217	102	18 241		44 287

* Recruitment incomplete at December 1976
  Data reproduced from Ref. 25

The pharmacological aspects of therapy are dealt with in detail in other chapters of this book and will not be referred to here except to emphasize that the physicians should be highly competent in the use of the various agents available. The importance of compliance has also been dealt with in detail (Chapter 7) and it only remains to emphasize the importance of this aspect of the programme and the fact that the difference between a cost-effective programme and a futile one may well depend on the compliance of the patients involved, which in turn will depend on the attention that is given to the matter by the physicians in charge.

Measurement of blood pressure
The lynch-pin of a community programme is the definition of blood pressure which is not only indicative of serious hypertensive complications in a situation where the probability of complications increases continuously as pressures rise, even in the normal range, but the identification of pressure at which pharmacological therapy will reduce complications on a significant scale. As well as defining such a cut-off point it is necessary in a community programme to establish methods of measuring it reproducibly. The variability of blood pressure recorded in an individual is well known. It has been analysed by Rose, Holland and Crowley[29], and Figure 5 from their paper summarizes the sources of variation. To some extent the variability is artefactual, depending on the accuracy of the sphygmomanometer and the accuracy and consistency of the observer, and the comparability of techniques if more than one observer is concerned.

Choice of instrument and reproducibility of measurements
Choice of reliable instruments and a programme of observer training are important in the initial planning of a screening project. The methods are discussed fully by Rose and Blackburn[30]. The cuff bladder size (at least 12 × 24 cm), the positioning of the cuff, rate of fall of mercury column of 2 mm/s, free access of stethoscope to the auscultation site, careful pinpointing of auscultation end-point read to the nearest 2 mm, avoidance of digit preference, having the subject seated with arm horizontal and relaxed and a preliminary period of rest for the subject are all important. The use of zero muddler[31] or other form of 'blind' recording sphygmomanometer such as the London School of Hygiene machine[29] are helpful in eliminating some aspects of observer error. The use of automated machines may also be considered, but careful evaluation of their accuracy should be made[32]. The use of training tapes[33] or films, both for training and testing of observers, is recommended.

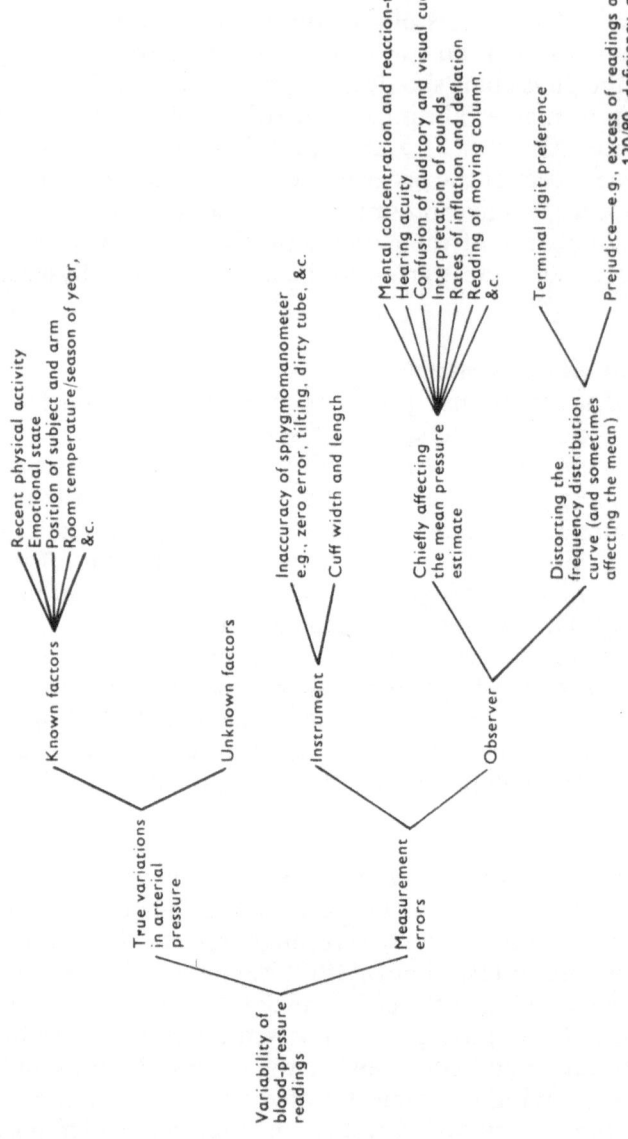

Figure 5 A schematic representation of some sources of variation in measuring blood pressure. From Ref. 29

Variability of blood pressure

More difficult to control is the variance within subjects which depends on physiological factors which vary with time. This form of variance was analysed by Armitage and Rose[34] and Armitage *et al.*[35], who showed that it could be greatly reduced by taking repeated measurements, both at a visit and on repeated visits. In a laboratory study in 10 subjects, in whom measurements were made repeatedly over a 6-week period, there was considerable random variation within the subjects which accounted for half of the standard deviation between them, both for systolic and diastolic pressures. As well as random variations there were also consistent trends with time. There was a fall (mean 3.06 mmHg) in systolic pressure from the first to the second readings at a visit, but no such change, in fact a slight rise (0.4 mmHg) for diastolic pressure (phase 5). However there was a highly significant downward trend for diastolic pressures on successive visits, with a mean fall of 8 mmHg from the first to the fourth visit and of 12 mmHg by the twentieth visit. Similar but larger variations were found in a field study in 722 subjects followed over 4 years. The authors concluded that repeated measurements at repeated visits increased the precision of blood pressure estimation very greatly. They concluded that in the field study, variations of blood pressure between subjects would be 16% greater systolic and 30% greater diastolic if a single estimation was used rather than readings on four separate occasions.

Similar variations have been reported by other investigators. Prineas *et al.*[36] observed a mean fall of 3.19 mmHg systolic and 0.56 mmHg diastolic between a first and second reading, a rise of 1.95 mmHg systolic and fall of 6.91 mmHg diastolic between visits 6 days apart. Hamilton *et al.*[9] noted a downward trend in repeated readings. In the screening phase of the Australian National Blood Pressure Study[37] there was a fall of 2.21 mmHg in mean systolic pressure and a slight rise (0.28 mmHg) in mean diastolic pressure between the first and second readings at the initial visit in 37 899 untreated subjects. However, taking the mean of two readings on a second visit 1–2 weeks later in 5 391 subjects who were hypertensive at the first visit, there was a mean fall of 6.54 mmHg systolic and 7.66 mmHg diastolic (see Tables 9 and 10).

Value of repeated visits

Thus, although it was apparent from the various reports from life insurance data that a single casual blood pressure reading was predictive of prognosis, definitive blood pressure levels and thus presumably prediction can be greatly refined by repeated readings, and any community programme must be based on such an approach.

Table 9 Australian national blood pressure study. Blood pressure (mmHg) of 37 899 untreated subjects attending primary screening

	Systolic (mean ± SD)	Diastolic (mean ± SD)
1st reading	137·92 ± 23·09	82·01 ± 13·42
2nd reading	135·71 ± 22·03	82·29 ± 13·05
Mean	136·82 ± 22·07	82·15 ± 12·84
Difference (1–2)	2·21 ± 9·39	−0·28 ± 6·43

Data reproduced from Ref. 37.

Table 10 Australian national blood pressure study. Blood pressure (mmHg) of 5391 untreated hypertensives at primary (S1) and secondary (S2) screenings

	Systolic (mean ± SD)	Diastolic (mean ± SD)
S1 (mean of 2 readings)	163·43 ± 20·36	102·37 ± 7·45
S2 (mean of 2 readings)	156·89 ± 21·92	94·71 ± 11·65
Mean (S1 + S2)/2	160·16 ± 19·41	98·53 ± 8·22
Difference (S1–S2)	6·54 ± 16·82	7·66 ± 10·59

Data reproduced from Ref. 37.

It is likely that guidelines for community programmes will in the future be based on the results of the therapeutic trials either presently completed or currently in progress[25], and as thése will give their results primarily (though not only) in terms of blood pressure levels it would seem sensible that the methods used in community programmes should be based on similar procedures (see Table 7). It will be noted that almost invariably these studies have used diastolic pressure phase 5 as the primary index and the lower cut-off point has been almost invariably 90 or 95 mmHg. All of them have required at least two visits and at least two readings at each visit, and all of them compute the definitive pressure as the mean of at least four readings. By contrast, many of the classic prevalence studies of the past have depended on single readings at one visit.

Although there has been constant search for parameters of blood pressure which are more highly predictive of prognosis than the simple systolic or diastolic pressure, at present this has been unsuccessful. A detailed analysis of the Framingham data[38] showed a stronger association of systolic than diastolic pressure with risk of coronary heart disease, but neither systolic nor diastolic measurement in combination, nor the pulse pressure nor the systolic lability independent of level of pressure, were more powerful in predicting subsequent onset of disease. Morris[39] concluded that elevated systolic pressure was more highly correlated with subsequent ischaemic heart disease than diastolic pressure, but blood pressure taken at rest, after mild exercise and various combinations of systolic or diastolic readings together were not more powerful in predicting ischaemic heart disease than the casual systolic or diastolic reading alone.

Implicit in a community control programme is that large numbers of individuals must be processed and large numbers of blood pressure measurers will be necessary. The logistics of the matter require therefore that the procedure must be as rapid and convenient as is consistent with the principles outlined above. A minimum regime, however, should include a blood pressure based on the mean of four readings taken on two separate occasions, with the patient seated for a reasonable period in a comfortable environment.

APPROACHES TO SCREENING

Within the usual medical services

There is great advantage in having hypertension diagnosed initially by the doctor who will be responsible for continuing care. The initial advice that hypertension is suspected, the arrangement for follow-up visit and confirmation and the smooth transition through initiation and stabilization of drug therapy and long-term management can develop with minimal psychic trauma or risk that the patient will default. It is in these early stages that patient understanding and attitudes are moulded and the seeds of compliance and adherence to therapy sown. In those communities where patient–doctor contacts are frequent, including both private and hospital visits, such a programme can cover a very large proportion of the community. This is especially so if it is supplemented by a community education campaign urging individuals who have not had their blood pressure taken recently to make a special visit to their doctor, and a professional education campaign urging doctors and hospitals to routinely measure pressures regardless of the reason for the patient's visit. Lovell *et al.*[40] found that 82% of the population aged 53–64 in a rural city in Australia contacted their doctors in a year, and that 66% of those attending had a blood pressure measurement. The additional measurements required for all patients who attend, and the further measurements on top of this to cope with the reviewing of all patients should they attend, was calculated to be approximately 150 per doctor per year. This did not seem to place too onerous a burden on the doctor's resources, a burden in any case which could be greatly lightened if the doctor's nurse or receptionist were trained to measure blood pressures.

Need for organized effort

To be effective such an approach to community-wide screening must be undertaken as a positive and definitive measure. Taking of blood pressure as a matter of mindless routine without purposive follow-on will achieve little. A sobering study of the matter was reported by Heller and Rose[41,42] which must reflect circumstances which are more often the rule than the exception. Analysis was made of 1784 new patients in either in-patient or out-patient clinics in two London hospitals. Only 58% of these had blood pressure recorded and of the 144 found hypertensive (systolic blood pressure 160 mmHg or more, diastolic 100 mmHg or more) a repeat reading was made in only 62% and only 12% went on to hypotensive therapy. In a random sample of 669 patients in seven general practices, only 24% had a blood pressure reading in 5 years. Hypertension was recorded in 74 of these patients but a repeat reading was made in only 61% of them. A total of 38% had been started on treatment, though only half of the latter were on treatment at the time of the survey.

The National Heart Foundation of Australia has based its community programme in hypertension control on the principle of identification of patients by routine measurements at doctor visits, and has conducted a continuing community education programme in press, radio and television urging a visit to the doctor for blood pressure measurement. At the same time it has written personally to doctors and hospital management urging that the opportunity be taken at all patient visits to ensure that blood pressure has been measured and that follow-up action is taken where appropriate[43].

Mass screening
An alternative approach to the identification of hypertensives is the mass community screening programme in one form or another. Such programmes are inexpensive and successful in finding hypertensives. They have been conducted in many areas throughout Australia, usually on the initiative of local doctors and frequently in association with service groups such as Rotary, Lions or Apex Clubs. Sited in public places or a hospital, they are particularly successful in specially designed and prominently decorated caravans or buses. The latter technique was used for the screening of 103 000 subjects to recruit subjects for the Australian National Blood Pressure Study[20]. Siting the vehicle in a busy shopping area, the use of media publicity, the publicized attendance of prominent citizens, and activities to win the support of medical practitioners in the area, were all aids to the success of such a programme.

Costs of mass screening
Trained screeners with no medical qualifications can be used successfully. The training should include the use of training tapes and films,

and personal training and testing by qualified personnel. The cost of screening, together with the cost of other aspects of an organized programme of hypertension control based on the experience of the Australian National Blood Pressure Study, is shown in Tables 11 and 12. The data on the cost of drugs derived from records of the Government Pharmaceutical Benefits Scheme in Australia are a realistic estimate of the total cost to the community in the years shown. The estimate of mass screening costs is based on the actual costs of screening the first 50 000 subjects in the Australian National Blood Pressure Study. The estimate of cost of medical care is based on the annual actual cost of supervising some 2000 patients in the same study.

Table 11 Cost of drugs used in Australia for treatment of hypertension (Australian dollars)

	1972	*1973*
Methyldopa	7 977 849	8 649 422
Debrisoquine	806 388	1 055 986
Guanethidine	2 372 676	2 220 660
Rauwolfia	1 078 902	1 061 508
Diuretics (50%)	5 255 330	5 943 081
Beta antagonists (20%)	179 805	404 949
	17 570 950	19 335 606

Data reproduced from Ref. 18.

Table 12 Estimated cost of treating all hypertensives in Australia (Australian dollars)

	Total cost	*Cost per head of population*	*Cost per hypertensive patient*
Screening	4 601 500	.61	3.74
Medical care	45 517 300	6.03	37.00
Drugs	44 075 800	5.84	35.81
TOTAL	94 194 600	12.48	76.55

Pitfalls to be avoided

In spite of the obvious attractions of mass screening there are certain pitfalls which must be carefully considered. Numerous studies have shown that the initial readings are likely to overestimate the subject's true pressure. Facilities for follow-up measurements in patients found to have high levels should therefore be ensured. Patients should not be advised that they are hypertensive on the basis of the first reading. Where suspected hypertensives are referred to their own doctors, there is a danger that on finding a lower and perhaps normal level on the second reading the doctor will be uncomplimentary, and if this occurs too frequently the whole procedure is brought into disrepute. To avoid this care should be taken to enlist the cooperation of the local medical profession where such a screening is to be conducted.

Stress has been laid on the likelihood that patients identified as hypertensive at the mass screening will not present themselves for the second reading as advised. Much will depend, however, on the procedures and relationships established. In the Australian National Blood Pressure Study, 989 subjects were identified in 85 583 screened, whose pressures were above the 'mild' cut-off point and thus were ineligible for the therapeutic trial. They were referred to their own doctors, and assessment of their responses was made subsequently. Information was obtained on the responses of 87·5% of them and in this group 91% did in fact consult a doctor[44].

Of great importance in the conducting of a mass screening programme is the follow-up of individuals found to have apparently dangerously high levels of blood pressure. Having offered such a programme to the community, it is the moral responsibility of the organizers to take all possible steps to ensure that these patients take follow-up measures. Enquiries should be made both to such patients and the doctors, after an appropriate interval, as to whether action has been taken.

'Do-it-yourself' screening

Relevant to the mass screening issue is the recent trend to retailing of do-it-yourself sphygmomanometers. The proposition is that individuals can buy a sphygmomanometer across the counter for approximately $30 in Australia, complete with instructions, and screen their own blood pressure and presumably that of family and friends. One can see no justification in terms of economics or convenience for such a procedure, and there are overwhelming probabilities of false-positive or false-negative results to the great harm of the subjects in either case. While self-measurement blood pressure devices can be valuable aids in the doctor's management of his hypertensive patient there can be no justification for this approach to the identification of hypertension in the community, and the same comments must apply to the coin-in-slot machines which I understand are installed in shopping areas in some countries. Fortunately these have not appeared in Australia.

INVESTIGATION OF PRIMARY CAUSE

Having identified a high proportion of hypertensives in a community, by whatever means, policy must be determined in respect to investigation for a primary cause. Obesity should be reduced, and the taking of oral contraceptives stopped. There is now general agreement that, in the absence of any clear pointers arising from the routine clinical examination, including ausculation, fundoscopy, urinalysis and chest X-ray, the sophisticated and demanding special biochemical and radiological investigations for renovascular and hormonal disorders are not warranted in a general community programme. However, in all cases the physician must be guided by his clinical judgment, and certainly serious consideration should be given to special investigations in young patients. The matter is dealt with in a report of the Intersociety Commission for Heart Disease Resources[45].

For the great majority of patients it is reasonable to commence surveillance and/or hypotensive therapy according to the indications of blood pressure level, presence of target organ damage, presence of risk factors and other features. For those subjects in whom control is difficult, or in whom specific indications arise during the course of subsequent supervision, special investigations may be reconsidered.

OBSERVATION OR PHARMACOLOGICAL THERAPY?

Moderate and severe hypertension

For patients with moderate or severe hypertension, or with target organ damage already apparent, the therapeutic trials referred to above, and particularly that of the Veterans Administration Cooperative Study, provide clear-cut indications that pharmacological therapy should be started at once. The evidence from these studies suggests that, provided the pressures are consistent and confirmed over a number of examinations, a diastolic pressure of 110 mmHg or greater, or systolic of 200 mmHg or greater require pharmacological treatment. Special consideration should be given to patients with high levels of other risk factors for coronary or cerebrovascular disease. It is of interest that, in the current studies, referred to in Tables 6 and 7, undertaken to investigate the appropriateness of therapy in lesser degrees of hypertension, a level of diastolic pressure between 105 and 115 mmHg (depending on the study) has been adopted as the cut-off point above which the case for pharmacological therapy is clearly established.

Mild hypertension

Until the results of these therapeutic trials in mild hypertension are available, the question of whether to start drug treatment for these lower levels of pressure must be left to the clinical judgment of the physician in charge of each patient, and will depend on his own appraisal of the relevant literature taken in conjunction with his confidence in the safety and effectiveness of drug treatment in his own hands, as well as the clinical profile of the patient.

The results of the first, and one of the smallest, of the therapeutic trials referred to, have now been published[46]. There were 389 subjects followed for an average of 7 years. Patients on active treatment were maintained at a blood pressure approximately 18 mmHg systolic and 11 mmHg diastolic lower than the controls. There was no statistically significant difference between the treated and control groups in terms of major hypertensive complications, although the trends were in favour of the treated group. There was a considerably lower incidence of cardiac enlargement and left ventricular hypertrophy by electrocardiographic evidence. The authors conclude that the study did not provide support for the use of pharmacological agents in mild hypertension. Full evaluation of the results must await comparison with the large studies still in progress.

More evidence needed in mild hypertension

It is certain that when these trials of drug therapy in mild hypertension reach acceptable conclusion there will still be a large group of borderline hypertensives in whom hypotensive drugs are not indicated, but who will require careful supervision in case pressures progress unfavourably. We know too little about the natural history of untreated mild hypertension, and it is anticipated that valuable information on this matter will also arise from the study of the control groups in the therapeutic trials referred to above.

Progression of mild hypertension

One of the very significant subgroups of control patients are those whose pressures rise above the upper cut-off point for mild hypertension. We look to the studies to indicate whether commencing pharmacological therapy at that time is adequate, or on the other hand too late, to prevent subsequent hypertensive complications. In the Australian National Blood Pressure Study, of some 2000 control subjects under observation for between 2 and 4 years, 172 have so far progressed to higher levels, requiring withdrawal from randomized treatment and institution of definitive therapy. As yet, detailed analysis of their characteristics has not been undertaken. The study of Miall and Chinn[47] among Welsh miners provides some indication of the rate of progression of hypertension among those initially at borderline or mild limits. In men of all ages, with initial diastolic blood pressure below 90 mmHg, only 3·8% had exceeded diastolic blood pressure of 109 mmHg at 15 years, and 5·1% of those with initial pressures below 100 mmHg. In women the figures were 5·5% and 7·3% respectively. The authors provide guidelines by age, sex and initial pressure for re-screening periods, to ensure that no more than 10% of hypertensives in a community requiring treatment, are not identified.

Trend of mild hypertension over time
Preliminary data from the control group of the Australian National Blood Pressure Study indicate that, on the average, blood pressures tend to fall over a period of several years' observation. The fall in pressure in the control subjects has been a surprising observation in a number of the therapeutic trials in mild hypertension[25,48,49] (see Figures 6 and 7). The reason for the fall in pressure is unclear at the present time. Some of it may be due to regression to the mean. Whether the regular periodic observation or the placebo tablets may also contribute is also undetermined. The possibility of a placebo effect was investigated in the Medical Research Council Therapeutic Trial in Mild Hypertension[48] in which

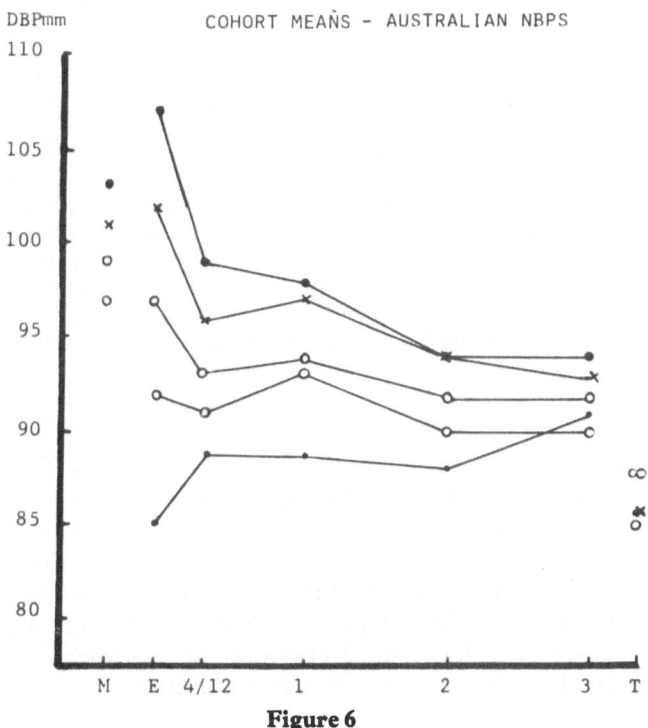

Figure 6

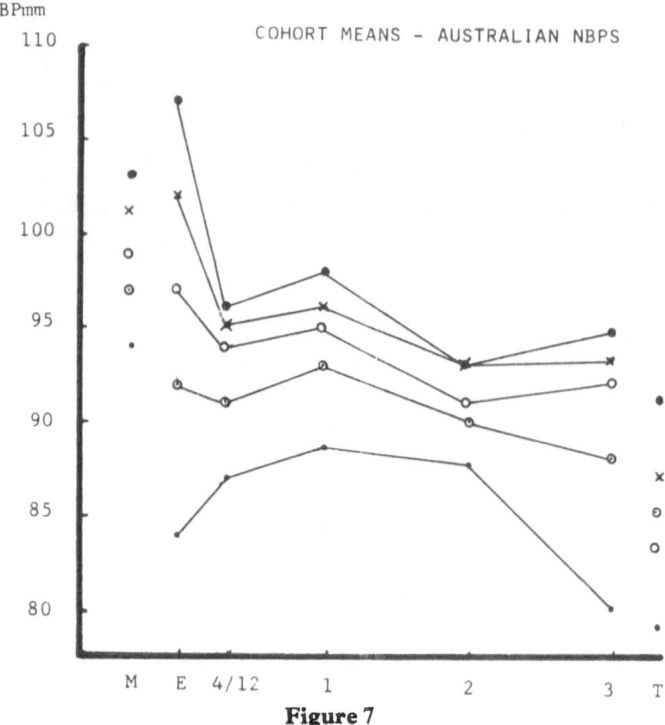

Figure 7

Figures 6 and 7　Diastolic blood pressure trends, men (Figure 6) and women (Figure 7). The cohorts are defined according to the mean pressures of two readings at the single visit immediately before instituting therapy as shown at the point E of the graph. The points shown at M refer to these cohorts and are based on the means of six readings at three visits prior to starting therapy. The numbers in each cohort of these control subjects vary from 150 to 250 men and 90 to 140 women. The values shown at M are also applicable to similar cohorts of the treated group. The point at T indicates the mean pressures at 3 years for the equivalent cohorts in the treated group, but it should be emphasized that the numbers at 3 years follow-up are small, varying from 15 to 35 subjects in both treated and controls. From Ref. 25

a subgroup of controls who attended clinics at the same frequency, but were taking no placebo tablets, showed changes in pressure identical to those found in patients who were receiving placebos. The phenomenon has considerable significance for those conducting community programmes, for it can be confidently anticipated that many subjects screened initially as mildly hypertensive will be found, during subsequent surveillance, to have blood pressures falling towards, or actually at, normal levels in the absence of hypotensive drugs.

EDUCATION AND A COMMUNITY PROGRAMME

Although, as stated above, there has been considerable reduction in morbidity and mortality from high blood pressure as a result of routine medical practices, it is also clear that these have not achieved the full potential that the pharmacological resources offer. It has been the experience of all those conducting community surveys that a great many patients known to be hypertensive are neither on therapy nor under surveillance, and many of those who are on hypotensive therapy do not have blood pressures under effective control.

Whether management of the patient with hypertension is by general practitioners, specialists, hospital-based clinic or some special community-based service, it is clear that much effort will be necessary to ensure a high standard of medical expertise and a high level of patient co-operation, and the health authorities must include in their overall strategy effective community and professional education programmes. The World Health Organization, the International Society and Federation of Cardiology, the National High Blood Pressure Education Program of the United States, and many other national bodies, are providing valuable guidelines and resource materials for such education programmes, and prior consultation with such organizations is recommended.

COMMUNITY PROGRAMMES AND PRIMARY PREVENTION

It was stated at the outset of this chapter that public health programmes involving screening and pharmacological therapy offer one of the greatest opportunities for medical intervention in our time. But control by drug therapy is a compromise and its benefits are qualified. Drug therapy carries with it risks of side-effects, high costs, and a lifetime of constraints for the patient. The real goal in control of hypertension is primary prevention, and the road to that goal is by elucidation of its mechanisms. A community control programme offers unparalleled opportunities for the investigation of mechanisms of hypertension and of measures for primary prevention in the large numbers of subjects concerned. The approaches to primary prevention have been discussed in the opening chapter of this book, and it is fitting to conclude on the note that it is the opportunity and duty of the authorities responsible for community control to foster research in conjunction with their programmes and to devote effort, funds and resources to that end.

References

1 Society of Actuaries (1959). *Build and Blood Pressure Study.* (Chicago)
2 Kannel, W. B., Schwartz, M. J. and McNamara, P. M. (1969). Blood pressure and risk of coronary heart disease: the Framingham Study. *Dis. Chest,* **56,** 43
3 Kannel, W. B., Wolf, P. S., Verter, J. and McNamara, P. M. (1970). Epidemiologic assessment of the role of blood pressure in stroke. *J. Amer. Med. Ass.,* **214,** 301
4 Paul, O. (1971). Risks of mild hypertension. A ten year report. *Brit. Heart J.,* **33** (Suppl.), 116
5 Janeway, T. C. (1913). A clinical study of hypertensive cardiovascular disease. *Arch. Intern. Med.,* **12,** 755
6 May, O. (1925). Mortality in relation to hyperpiesia. *Brit. Med. J.,* **2,** 1166
7 United States Public Health Service. (1966). Hypertension and hypertensive heart disease in adults. *National Center for Health Statistics,* Series **11,** no. 13
8 Boe, J., Humerfelt, S. and Wedervang, F. (1957). The blood pressure in a population. *Acta Med. Scand.,* **321** (Suppl.), 1
9 Hamilton, M., Pickering, G. W., Roberts, J. A. F. and Sowry, G. S. C. (1954). Arterial pressure in a population. (i) The arterial pressure in a general population. *Clin. Sci.,* **13,** 11
10 McCall, M. G., Kelsall, R. G., Rosman, D. L., Stenhouse, N. S. and Welborn, T. A. (1973). Blood pressure in Busselton, Western Australia. *Med. J. Aust.,* **2** (suppl), 8
11 Wilber, J. A. (1967). Detection and control of hypertensive disease in Georgia, USA. In J. Stamler, R. Stamler and T. N. Pullman (eds.). *The Epidemiology of Hypertension* (New York: Grune and Stratton)
12 Leishman, A. W. D. (1963). Merits of reducing high blood pressure. *Lancet,* **1,** 1284
13 Hamilton, M., Thompson, E. N. and Wisniewski, T. K. M. (1964). The role of blood pressure control in preventing complications of hypertension. *Lancet,* **1,** 235
14 Marshall, J. F. (1964). A trial of long term hypotensive therapy in cerebrovascular disease. *Lancet,* **1,** 10
15 Wolff, F. W. and Lindeman, R. D. (1966). Effects of treatment in hypertension. Results of a controlled study. *J. Chron. Dis.,* **19,** 227
16 Veterans Administration Cooperative Study Group (1967). Effects of treatment on morbidity in hypertension: results in patients with diastolic blood pressure averaging 115 through 129 mmHg. *J. Amer. Med. Ass.,* **202,** 1028
17 Moriyama, I. M., Krueger, D. E. and Stamler, J. (1971). *Cardiovascular Diseases in the United States of America.* (Boston: Harvard University Press)
18 Reader, R. (1975). Hypertension and the community. *Acta Med. Scand.,* **576** (Suppl.), 83
19 Paul, O. (1974). A survey of the epidemiology of hypertension, 1964–74. *Mod. Concepts Cardiovasc. Dis.,* **43,,** 99
20 Abernethy, J. D. (1974). The Australian National Blood Pressure Study. *Med. J. Aust.,* **1,** 821
21 Prineas, R. J., Stephens, W. B. and Lovell, R. R. (1973). Blood pressure and its treatment in a community. The Albury Blood Pressure Study. *Med. J. Aust.,* **1,** 5
22 Veterans Administrative Cooperative Study Group (1970). Effects of treatment on morbidity in hypertension: results in patients with diastolic blood pressure averaging 90 through 114 mmHg. *J. Amer. Med. Ass.,* **213,** 1143
· 23 Veterans Administrative Cooperative Study Group (1972). Effects of treatment on morbidity in hypertension: influence of age, diastolic pressure and prior cardiovascular disease: further analysis of side effects. *Circulation,* **45,** 991

24 World Health Organization. (1975). Effectiveness of treatment in mild forms of hypertension. *Report of a Joint WHO–ISH Meeting, Madrid*, CVD.75.5

25 Reader, R. (1977). Therapeutic trials in mild hypertension ongoing throughout the world. *Ann. N.Y. Acad. Sci.* (In press)

26 Finnerty, F. A., Mattie, E. C. and Finnerty, Francis A. (1973). Hypertension in the inner city. (i) Analysis of clinic dropouts. *Circulation*, **47**, 73

27 Wilber, J. A. and Barrow, J. G. (1972). Hypertension, a community problem. *Amer. J. Med.*, **52**, 653

28 Sacket, D. (1974). Screening for disease: cardiovascular diseases. *Lancet*, **2**, 1189

29 Rose, G. A., Holland, W. W. and Crowley, E. A. (1964). A sphygmomanometer for epidemiologists. *Lancet*, **1**, 296

30 Rose, G. A. and Blackburn, H. (1968). Cardiovascular survey methods. *WHO, Monograph*, Series No. 56

31 Garrow, J. S. (1963). Zero muddler for unprejudiced sphygmomanometry. *Lancet*, **2**, 1205

32 Labarthe, D., Hawkins, C. M. and Remington, R. D. (1973). Evaluation of performance of selected devices for measuring blood pressure. *Amer. J. Cardiol.*, **32**, 546

33 Rose, G. (1965). Standardisation of observers in blood pressure measurement. *Lancet*, **1**, 673

34 Armitage, P. and Rose, G. A. (1966). The variability of measurements of casual blood pressure. (i) A laboratory study. *Clin. Sci.*, **30**, 325

35 Armitage, P., Fox, W., Rose, G. A. and Tinker, C. M. (1966). The variability of measurements of casual blood pressure. (ii) Survey experience. *Clin, Sci.*, **30**, 337

36 Prineas, R. J., Stephens, W. B. and Lovell, R. R. (1973). Prevalence of hypertension and its treatment in an Australian community: implications for screening. *Singapore Med. J.*, **14**, 429

37 Reader, R. (1975). Screening methods in community control of hypertension. In G. Berglund, L. Hansson and L. Werko (eds.). *Pathophysiology and Management of Arterial Hypertension*, pp. 250–257. (Molndal, Sweden: A. Lindgren and Soner AB)

38 Kannel, W. B., Gordon, T. and Schwartz, M. J. (1971). Systolic versus diastolic blood pressure and risk of coronary heart disease. *Amer. J. Cardiol.*, **27**, 335

39 Morris, J. M., Kagan, A., Pattison, D. C., Gardner, M. J. and Raffle, P. A. B. (1966). Incidence and prediction of ischaemic heart disease in London busmen. *Lancet*, **2**, 553

40 Lovell, R. R., Stephens, W. B., Thompson, L. and Ulman, R. (1976). The rate of initiation of treatment for hypertension in a community, 1971–75. *Aust. NZ. J. Med.*, **6**, 398

41 Heller, R. F. and Rose, G. (1977). Current management of hypertension in hospital. *Brit. Med. J.*, **1**, 1441

42 Heller, R. F. and Rose, G. (1977). Current management of hypertension in general practice. *Brit. Med. J.*, **1**, 1442

43 Bauer, G. E. (1976). Correspondence. *Med. J. Aust.*, **2**, 466

44 Hunyor, S. N., Bauer, G. E., Abernethy, J. D., Baker, J. L., Bullen, M. U., Lamb, M. L. and Stewart M. R. (1977). Detection and follow-up of moderate and severe hypertensive subjects in the Australian community. *Med. J. Aust.*, **1**, 517

45 Intersociety Commission for Heart Disease Resources. (1972). Irvine S. Wright and Donald T. Fredrickson. (eds.) Guidelines for the detection, diagnosis and management of hypertensive populations. *Circulation*, **64**, A–263

46 Smith, W. M., Edlavitch, S. A. and Krushat, W. M. (1977). United States Public

Health Service Hospitals Intervention Trial in Mild Hypertension. *Proc. Hahnemann Medical Colleges Vth Annual Symposium on Hypertension,* Puerto Rico

47 Miall, W. E. and Chinn, S. (1974). Screening for hypertension: some epidemiological observations. *Brit. Med. J.,* **2,** 595

48 MRC Working Party. (1977). Randomised controlled trial of treatment for mild hypertension: design and pilot trial. *Brit. Med. J.,* **1,** 1437

49 World Health Organisation. (1977). Joint WHO–ISH Liaison Committee on mild hypertension trials. *Report of the 2nd meeting, New York, February, 1977.* CVD.77.2

3

Evaluation of the hypertensive patient

R. W. Gifford, Jr

INTRODUCTION

In the past, too much emphasis has been placed on the diagnostic aspects of hypertension and not enough attention has been given to the importance of therapy. Perhaps this is one reason why no more than 30% of hypertensives in the United States have their blood pressures adequately controlled.

Thirty years ago, when effective medical therapy for hypertension was non-existent, it was appropriate to subject patients to extensive diagnostic evaluations designed to uncover the few who might have a surgically remediable cause for their hypertension. Except for surgical sympathectomy, there was nothing else to do for them.

It is now apparent, however, that curable causes for hypertension are indeed rare (Table 1) and that more than 95% of hypertensive patients must be treated medically[1,2]. Moreover, there is no longer any doubt that antihypertensive therapy prolongs life and prevents or postpones the cardiovascular and renal complications of hypertension[3,4].

These developments, along with obvious limitations in manpower, facilities and economic resources, have led to a review of the traditional concepts of the routine evaluation of hypertension[5–10] and have brought into focus the need to simplify and streamline it, and make it more relevant to changing objectives.

Emphasis must be on those examinations which will immediately and materially influence decisions regarding urgency of therapy and choice of drugs. Confronted with a huge backlog of untreated hypertensive patients, it is imperative that more of our resources be devoted to the task of getting patients started on appropriate treatment after a minimal evaluation. If the hypertension then proves to be resistant to a good therapeutic regimen, a 'second look', with more detailed and elaborate diagnostic investigation, is indicated.

43

Table 1   Frequency of curable forms of hypertension encountered at the Mayo and Cleveland clinics

Curable causes	Mayo clinic [1] (80 000 patients)*		Cleveland clinic [2] (4939 patients)†	
	No.	Percentage	No.	Percentage
Primary aldosteronism	8	0·01	20	0·4
Phaeochromocytoma	31	0·04	9	0·18
Renal vascular disease (operated)	140	0·18	67	1·4
Coarctation of the aorta	NS	NS	30	0·6
Cushing's syndrome	NS	NS	11	0·2

* Estimated number of hypertensive patients seen at Mayo Clinic in 1973, 1974 and 1975 based on age- and sex-specific frequencies reported from US National Health Survey, 1960–62.

† No. of patients first given diagnosis of hypertension at Cleveland Clinic in 1966–67.

NS = not significant

WHOM, WHEN AND WHERE TO EVALUATE

Except in emergency situations when hypertension is severe, or complications are impending or present, treatment should be withheld until the diagnostic work-up is complete. If the patient is already on therapy, it is best to proceed with the history and physical examination before deciding on the advisability of, or even the necessity for, stopping it.

For patients with mild or borderline hypertension, it is reasonable to defer evaluation until a series of measurements confirm that the average blood pressure is elevated. The Hypertension Study Group of the Inter-Society Commission for Heart Disease Resources[9] has proposed that evaluation be carried out for persons less than 40 years of age who have blood pressures in excess of 140 mmHg systolic and/or 90 mmHg diastolic on at least two of the three determinations on different days. For patients older than this, the limits were 160 mmHg systolic and/or 95 mmHg diastolic on at least two of the three consecutive readings. For children less than 15 years of age, limits should be reduced.

For at least 90% of hypertensive patients, the pre-treatment evaluation can and should be carried out on an out-patient basis in the physician's office. Hospitalization is necessary only for those patients who have severe hypertension with impending or actual complications, or who require specialized diagnostic procedures that cannot be done on an out-patient basis.

OBJECTIVES OF THE PRE-TREATMENT EVALUATION

Objectives of the evaluation of hypertensive patients, as well as the minimal work-up that is needed to accomplish them, are listed in Table 2.

Table 2   Examinations indicated for every hypertensive patient and the objectives which they accomplish

Examination	*Evaluate target organs and estimate prognosis*	*Discover co-existing disease*	*Discover curable causes*	*Identification of other risk factors*
History and physical	+	+	+	+
Haemogram	−	+	−	−
Urinalysis	+	+	−	−
BUN and/or serum creatinine	+	−	−	−
Serum potassium	−	−	+	−
Serum cholesterol and triglycerides (for patients less than 60 years of age)	−	−	−	+
EKG	+	−	−	−

Evaluation of target organs and estimation of prognosis

Evaluation of the target organs of hypertension, the brain, eyes, heart and kidneys deserves high priority, because the presence of hypertensive complications has an important bearing on prognosis as well as on the choice of antihypertensive drugs and the urgency with which they are administered. This is probably the most important objective of the pre-treatment evaluation.

To discover co-existing disease

It is important to put the hypertension in perspective in the patient's total health picture. Sometimes other conditions or diseases are more important than, or should temporarily take precedence over, the hypertension. Co-existing diseases may influence the choice of antihypertensive drugs.

To discover curable causes

The importance of identifying potentially curable causes for hypertension should not be minimized, especially for young patients and for patients whose hypertension is resistant to a good medical regimen. Clues to the presence of curable hypertension can usually be obtained from the history, physical examination and the selected laboratory procedures listed in Table 2. It is unnecessary to mandate that all hypertensives should have rapid sequence intravenous urograms, tests for phaeochromocytoma, determinations of plasma renin activity and plasma or urinary aldosterone. Searching for curable causes when the preliminary evaluation affords no clues is unproductive, sometimes hazardous and adds unnecessarily to the cost of medical care.

Identifications of other risk factors

Control of hypertension has been shown to reduce the frequency of all of the complications of hypertension except for those due to coronary disease[3,4]. Because hypertension is only one of several risk factors for coronary atherosclerosis, it is possible that by identifying and simultaneously managing other risk factors the high incidence of death and disability from coronary disease in hypertensive patients will be favourably influenced.

To verify that hypertension is sustained

This objective is not shown in Table 2 because it is simply accomplished by repeated determinations of blood pressure. A minimum of three determinations of blood pressure should be made on separate visits before the decision is reached about the necessity for treatment, unless hypertension is severe and target organ damage is already evident. In patients with mild or borderline elevations of blood pressure, the decision about whether to proceed with further evaluation can be deferred until it has been established that the average diastolic and/or systolic blood pressures meet certain criteria outlined in the previous section.

Indications for home blood pressure recordings

When diastolic blood pressure is less than 104 mmHg on one or more occasions, I would prefer to have more than three readings before deciding about the necessity for therapy. In this situation, it has been my custom for a long time to lend a sphygmomanometer to patients who have borderline elevations, so that they can take their pressures at home every day for 1–3 weeks before I decide whether they need antiphypertensive drugs or even further evaluation.

In this regard it must be remembered that blood pressure measurements made while the patient is hospitalized are almost invariably lower than ambulatory pressures and should not be relied on when making a decision about the necessity for medical treatment.

THE BASIC EXAMINATIONS

The recommended basic examinations are listed in Table 2. These represent a consensus of the Inter-Society Commission on Heart Disease Resources[9], the Joint National Committee on Detection, Evaluation, and Treatment of High Blood Pressure[10] as well as my own modifications of these. The Inter-Society Commission on Heart Disease Resources and the Joint National Committee recommended only haematocrit (and not a complete blood count) and did not recommend routine microscopic examination of the urine, whereas it has been my practice to obtain a complete blood count and a complete urinalysis. The Joint National Committee recommendations do not include serum uric acid, blood glucose, serum cholesterol, serum triglycerides or chest X-ray, whereas the ICHD report recommends all of these with the exception of triglycerides. It has been my practice to include serum cholesterol and triglycerides only for patients less than 60 years of age, because available data indicate that after this age the blood lipids are not as important prognostically and that attempts to correct abnormalities do not influence atherosclerotic complications.

Since serum uric acid and blood glucose do not immediately influence the choice of antihypertensive drugs I do not include them as routine, although their inclusion could be justified on the basis of identification of other risk factors and evaluation of the patient's general health status.

These minor differences in opinion become moot because in most blood chemistry laboratories it is less expensive and more convenient to obtain the battery of 18 automated determinations than to order selectively the four or five that are specifically needed for the evaluation of the hypertensive patient.

It should be specifically pointed out that the rapid sequence intravenous urogram, tests for phaeochromocytoma and measurement of plasma renin activity are not included in the basic examination.

History and physical examination
The most important part of the evaluation is the history and physical examination. These can provide clues to the severity of hypertension, the presence of target organ involvement, and the presence of curable causes that cannot be obtained in any other way. Moreover, the absence of certain historical features or physical findings may make unnecessary an exhaustive search for some of the esoteric curable causes for hyperten-

sion. A thorough history and physical examination may reveal unsuspected and unrelated disease which may alter the prognosis and the approach to therapy. The importance of multiple determinations of blood pressure before deciding about the necessity for drug treatment has already been emphasized. It can be seen, therefore, that the history and physical examination are indispensable to all of the objectives of the pretreatment evaluation (Table 2).

History

While most patients with essential hypertension have a family history of hypertension, the presence or absence of a family history does not clearly discriminate between primary and secondary hypertension. Many patients do not know for certain what their relatives' blood pressures are, or they have the mistaken impression that stroke or heart attack is prima facie evidence that their relatives had hypertension and therefore, innocently, give a falsely positive response to this question. It is best to use the term 'high blood pressure' when interrogating a patient about family members because many lay persons believe that hypertension is synonymous with nervousness and excitability.

A family history of premature death or disability from stroke or heart attack is particularly ominous, and the more family members so affected (and the younger the age at which they were affected), the greater concern for the patient. This type of family history might be the deciding factor in the decision to treat patients with mild or borderline hypertension.

A history of acute glomerulonephritis, proteinuria, haematuria, recurrent urinary tract infections, renal colic, or renal trauma should make the physician suspect that the hypertension may be due to chronic renal disease, especially when it can be established that the urinary tract symptoms or abnormalities (especially proteinuria) preceded the onset of hypertension.

It is important to distinguish between duration and discovery of hypertension. Since hypertension is notoriously asymptomatic, it may have existed long before it was discovered. In obtaining a history, it is helpful to establish not only when the hypertension was first discovered but when the last previous normal blood pressure reading was obtained.

Abrupt onset of hypertension with rapid progression suggests renovascular disease. On the other hand, a long history of unusual lability of blood pressure that gradually progressed to sustained hypertension is characteristic of essential hypertension. Onset of sustained hypertension before the age of 25 years or after the age of 50 years should prompt the physician to suspect renovascular hypertension.

Women should be asked about the ingestion of oestrogen preparations, especially oral contraceptive agents which can precipitate or aggravate hypertension. The relationship between the onset of hypertension and the initiation of oestrogen therapy should be sought. It is quite likely that oral contraceptive therapy is the most frequent cause of curable hypertension in pre-menopausal women.

In the search for other risk factors, patients should be interrogated about their smoking and exercise habits. Cigarette smoking constitutes one of the most important risk factors in sudden death from coronary disease. The more cigarettes smoked per day, the greater risk. Sedentary individuals are at greater risk than those who exercise regularly.

A history of headache, excessive perspiration, palpitations and/or tachycardia, tremor, unusual anxiety, and episodic pallor of the face, suggest phaeochromocytoma, especially when symptoms occur paroxysmally in combination and are accompanied by recent weight loss. Other historical clues to phaeochromocytoma include paradoxical response to anti-hypertensive agents, hypertension precipitated by induction of anaesthesia and diabetes. In the absence of any of these historical features, it is not necessary to include tests for phaeochromocytoma in the evaluation of the hypertensive patient.

The patient should be questioned carefully for evidence of atherosclerotic complications, including transient ischaemic attacks, stroke, angina pectoris, myocardial infarction, or intermittent claudication – all of which compromise prognosis and often influence the choice of drugs.

Unusual exertional dyspnoea, orthopnoea, paroxysmal nocturnal dyspnoea, and pedal oedema provide evidence of heart failure which demands a prompt reduction of blood pressure in most instances.

It is helpful to obtain a history of antihypertensive drugs which have been prescribed previously. Particularly discouraging is a history of intolerance to all antihypertensive drugs, especially when the alleged side-effects are vague and much the same for each and every drug, bearing no relationship to their pharmacological action. Patients who relate this type of history usually experience similar adverse effects from placebo, and it is unlikely that an acceptable regimen can be established.

Physical examination
The physical examination of the hypertensive patient should be complete, with special attention to certain details that are particularly relevant to hypertensive cardiovascular disease.

Blood pressure measurement   Initially, the blood pressure should be measured in both arms after the patient has been supine for at least 5 min. If there is no significant difference between the two arms, it is unnecessary to measure the blood pressure in both arms thereafter. It is now generally accepted that the 5th Korotkoff phase (disappearance of sounds) should be used as the diastolic pressure, although both the 4th (muffling of sounds) and 5th phases should be recorded if there is more than a 5 mmHg disparity between the two. Blood pressure should also be measured after the patient has been standing for at least 2 min. Any disparity of 10 mmHg or more in systolic or diastolic blood pressure between the two arms should be confirmed by repeated measurements. If it is consistent, it more often signifies an occlusive atherosclerotic plaque in the subclavian artery, usually on the left. For follow-up purposes and evaluation of treatment the blood pressure should always be taken in the arm that gives the highest reading. In order to minimize falsely high readings in patients with obese arms, a cuff that is longer and wider (thigh cuff) than the standard cuff should be used.

Blood pressure measurements in the thigh are cumbersome and difficult to make, and are grossly inaccurate because of the large muscle mass in the thigh. Even a large cuff grossly overestimates blood pressure in the thigh, so that any reading equal to or less than the blood pressure recorded in the arm is abnormal and indicates obstructive disease in the aorta, iliac or femoral arteries proximally.

Ophthalmoscopic examination Ophthalmoscopic examination to classify the severity of hypertension is one of the most important parts of evaluation of the hypertensive patient, because it provides information relative to prognosis that is not obtainable in any other way[11]. The Keith–Wagener–Barker classification of hypertension based solely on ophthalmoscopic findings is outlined in Table 3. In general, spasm of

Table 3 Ophthalmoscopic classification of hypertension (Keith–Wagener–Barker)

		Retinal arterioles			
Group	Sclerosis	General spasm	Haemor-rhages	Exu-dates	Papill-oedema
I	−	+	−	−	−
II	+	+	±	−	−
III	±	+	+	+	−
IV	±	+	±	±	+

− = absent
+ = present
± = present or absent

the retinal arterioles is related to the level of diastolic blood pressure while sclerosis (heightened light reflex, arteriovenous nicking) of the retinal arterioles is a reflection of duration of hypertension. Consequently, the finding of severe arteriolar spasm, focal and generalized, with little or no sclerosis (arteriospastic angiography) is suggestive of recent onset of severe hypertension and is a clue to the presence of renovascular disease, phaeochromocytoma or some other form of secondary hypertension. On the other hand, severe arteriolosclerosis with mild spasm suggests chronic hypertension of mild or moderate severity, more compatible with primary hypertension. The presence of retinal haemorrhages and exudates with papilloedema (group IV), or without papilloedema (group III) is a sign of accelerated hypertension and constitutes a quasi-emergency. The term 'malignant hypertension' should be reserved for Keith–Wagener–Barker group IV (papilloedema).

Minimal or no constriction and sclerosis of the retinal arterioles is reassuring, because this usually means that hypertension is labile even though one or more casual readings have been alarmingly high.

Microemboli in the retinal arterioles usually indicate that there is an ulcerated plaque in the internal carotid artery on the side of the microemboli. Frequently, but by no means always, patients who have retinal micro-emboli also have symptoms of transient ischaemic attacks.

Cardiac examination Of the three target organs of hypertension, the heart is more frequently affected clinically than the brain or kidneys. Not only does hypertension accelerate coronary atherosclerosis, leading to an increased incidence of atherosclerotic heart disease in hypertensive compared to normotensive patients, but it also affects the left ventricle directly, leading to hypertrophy with ultimate dilation and failure (hypertensive heart disease). The earliest physical sign of cardiac involvement is the presence of a 4th heart sound (atrial gallop). This is usually audible before there is any detectable cardiac enlargement and before there are physical signs of increased left ventricular thrust against the precordium, both in amplitude and duration. The 4th heart sound correlates well with the P-wave abnormality on the electrocardiogram. A 3rd heart sound (ventricular gallop) is usually a late manifestation of hypertensive heart disease and heralds the onset of left ventricular failure with moist rales in both lung bases. When the right heart also fails there is hepatomegaly, jugular venous distension and pedal oedema.

When hypertension is severe a decrescendo diastolic murmur may be heard in the second right interspace and along the left sternal border, indicative of relative aortic insufficiency. If this murmur does not disappear when hypertension is successfully treated the physician should suspect that it is due to intrinsic disease of the aortic valve or its ring.

The syndrome of hyperkinetic circulation ('hyperdynamic heart') usually occurs in adolescents and young adults, and is characterized by labile, predominantly systolic hypertension, resting tachycardia, a hyperactive precordium due to increase in left ventricular contractility, prominent pulsations in the carotid arteries and a systolic 'flow' murmur heard best along the left sternal border.

Examination of the peripheral arteries   Special attention should be given to the examination of the peripheral vascular system, looking for evidence of occlusive disease, bruits, and aneurysms. The incidence of atherosclerotic occlusive arterial disease of the carotid–subclavian–vertebral systems and the aorta–iliac–femoral systems is increased in hypertensives. Aneurysms, especially of the abdominal aorta, are more frequently found in hypertensive than in normotensive individuals, and the prognosis is worse for hypertensives.

In addition to careful palpation of the peripheral arteries, the physician should listen for bruits over the carotid arteries in the neck, the subclavian arteries in the supraclavicular spaces, the abdominal aorta and renal arteries, and the femoral arteries in the groin.

The presence of a diastolic component to the bruit and/or a thrill palpable over a peripheral artery is indicative of a tight stenosis.

A systolic–diastolic bruit in the epigastrium or in one or both upper quadrants of the abdomen is so suggestive of renal artery stenosis that renal angiography is indicated even if the rapid sequence intravenous urogram is normal, provided that the patient is a candidate for corrective surgery. On the other hand, systolic bruits without diastolic components have no particular significance in the abdomen. A systolic bruit over the carotid, however, may be quite significant.

A systolic bruit over the femoral artery in the groin signifies atherosclerotic disease of the aorta and/or the ipsilateral iliac artery, but it does not necessarily indicate that it is occlusive.

When pulses in the lower extremities are absent, impaired or delayed in a hypertensive child, adolescent or young adult, coarctation of the aorta should be a prime diagnostic consideration.

Neurological examination   Gross neurological deficits are not likely to be overlooked, but more subtle deficits suggesting old cerebral infarcts which may not have been diagnosed clinically should be sought.

Abdominal examination   Palpable enlargement of one or both kidneys should make the examiner suspect polycystic renal disease, hydronephrosis, or renal tumour. Rarely, a phaeochromocytoma is large enough to be palpable but adrenal cortical adenomas causing primary aldosteronism are never palpable.

General observations Tremor, tachycardia, restlessness, and excessive perspiration can be manifestations of phaeochromocytoma, or the syndrome of hyperdynamic circulation, as well as anxiety, hyperthyroidism, and chronic alcoholism. Truncal obesity, frontal baldness, prominent striae and atrophy of the skin with spontaneous ecchymoses are clues to the diagnosis of Cushing's syndrome.

Laboratory and roentgenographic examinations
Routine tests
Haemogram, urinalysis, serum creatinine or BUN Although a high haematocrit is sometimes the clue to the presence of renovascular hypertension[12], the main purpose of the haemogram in the evaluation of the hypertensive patient is to assess the patient's general health status.

Urinalysis, serum creatinine and/or BUN are included to evaluate the kidney as a target or inciting organ in hypertension. If the urinalysis is negative (including microscopic examination) it is unlikely that the hypertension is due to primary renal disease. If the urinalysis is abnormal, the clinician must attempt to determine whether the abnormality is a primary event, secondary to longstanding hypertension (nephrosclerosis) or unrelated to the hypertension.

Serum potassium The serum potassium concentration is a clue to the presence of primary aldosteronism. A normal serum potassium concentration rules out primary aldosteronism except in patients on very low sodium diets. By assuring that the patient has even an average sodium chloride intake for 2 or 3 days before blood for the serum potassium determination is drawn, this pitfall can be avoided. The serum potassium determination also serves as a baseline for subsequent thiazide therapy. Diuretic-induced hypokalaemia may persist for as long as 6 weeks after stopping therapy, but diuretic-induced kaliuresis rarely lasts longer than 48 hours after stopping therapy. Consequently, further investigation is indicated whenever inappropriate kaliuresis (> 40 mEq/24 h) accompanies hypokalaemia ($< 3 \cdot 5$ mEq/l) provided that a diuretic has not been administered within the previous 72 h.

Serum cholesterol and triglycerides Determinations of serum cholesterol and triglycerides are important because hyperlipidaemia is an additional risk factor for coronary disease.

Electrocardiogram The electrocardiogram is included to evaluate the heart as a target organ. The first electrocardiographic manifestation of hypertensive heart disease is the P-wave abnormality manifested by biphasic P-waves in V-1 and broad, notched P-waves in the left precordial leads. As left ventricular hypertrophy progresses, there is increased amplitude of the R-waves and finally, ST-T abnormalities appear. The electrocardiogram is also helpful in identifying patients who have had a previous myocardial infarction, even though there is no good clinical history for it.

Special tests
Examinations which have not been recommended for the routine evaluation of the hypertensive patient include the rapid sequence intravenous urogram, tests for phaeochromocytoma, serum uric acid and blood glucose and plasma renin activity.

Rapid sequence intravenous pyelogram   The indications for obtaining a rapid sequence intravenous pyelogram as part of the evaluation of the hypertensive patient are listed in Table 4. The younger the patient, and the more severe the hypertension, the more important it is to make the

Table 4   Some indications for rapid sequence intravenous pyelogram (hypertensive IVP) in the diagnosis of hypertension*

Systolic/diastolic bruit in abdomen†
Age $\leqslant$ 30 yrs and diastolic blood pressure $\geqslant$ 110 mmHg
Diastolic blood pressure $\geqslant$ 130 mmHg at any age
Premalignant or malignant (group III or IV) hypertension
Hypertension resistant to treatment
Urological indications‡ (history of calculi, haematuria, recurrent urinary tract infections, obstructive symptoms; pyuria, haematuria, cylindruria, azotaemia)

* It is unnecessary and inappropriate to perform IVP or renal angiography looking for renovascular disease if the patient is not a candidate for surgical treatment should a lesion be found.
† Systolic bruits have no diagnostic significance.
‡ Irrespective of blood pressure.

diagnosis of renovascular hypertension because the cure rate is high when renal vein renin activity lateralizes to the suspect side in patients with fibrous disease of the renal artery. On the other hand, the surgical cure rate is no better than 50% and the mortality rate in some series exceeds 5% for older patients with atherosclerotic renovascular disease; consequently, it is hardly worth the effort to identify such patients unless hypertension is resistant to a good medical regimen. For this reason there are many physicians who do not advise a routine hypertensive intravenous pyelogram in patients older than 30 or 40 years unless hypertension is severe or resistant to therapy. While there are many clues to the presence of renovascular hypertension (Table 5), it can be asymptomatic, can occur at any age, and can present as insidiously as essential hypertension without a systolic–diastolic bruit in the abdomen. Moreover, the rapid sequence intravenous pyelogram is normal in approximately 17% of patients who are subsequently cured by surgery[13], so if clinical suspicion is strong a renal angiogram should be performed without a preliminary rapid sequence intravenous pyelogram.

Table 5 Clinical clues to the diagnosis of renovascular hypertension

Abrupt onset or exacerbation of hypertension with rapid progression
Onset of hypertension before age 30 or after age 50
Systolic and diastolic bruit in epigastrium and/or upper quadrant
Accelerated hypertension (group III or IV, Keith–Wagener–Barker)
Arteriospastic retinal vascular changes with little or no sclerosis (arteriospastic angiopathy)
Abnormal rapid sequence intravenous pyelogram (disparity in appearance time or density of contrast medium or in size of kidneys)

If hypertension has existed for more than 5 years, it is unlikely that nephrectomy or renal revascularization will relieve it, especially if the rapid sequence intravenous pyelogram is normal[14]. Consequently, the identification of patients with renovascular disease who have had hypertension for a long time is not so important, unless there has been recent exacerbation of their disease.

Once renovascular disease has been identified on the renal angiogram, it is important to establish its pathophysiological significance by measurements of renal vein renin activity before considering surgical treatment. The ideal situation is one in which the renal vein renin activity from the involved kidney is definitely higher than normal and at least 1·5 times that from the opposite, uninvolved kidney. The renal vein renin activity from the uninvolved kidney should be equal to or less than peripheral venous or aortic blood renin activity, indicating that its renin secretion has been suppressed. The predictability of renal vein renin measurements can be enhanced by stimulating the renin–angiotensin system with a very low sodium diet and/or administration of a diuretic before blood is obtained.

Serum uric acid and blood glucose Because I do not consider that elevations of serum uric acid or blood glucose constitute contraindications to the use of thiazide diuretics, the main purpose for obtaining these examinations is to evaluate the patient's general health status, and because hyperuricaemia and hyperglycaemia increase risk of atherosclerotic complications. However, there is no evidence that correcting these abnormalities lessens the risk.

Roentgenogram of the chest   There is not unanimous agreement that roentgenogram of the chest is a necessary part of the pre-treatment evaluation of the hypertensive patient. Cardiomegaly detected by roentgenogram of the chest is usually not apparent until after there is EKG evidence of left ventricular hypertrophy, so that the main justification for including it would be as part of the evaluation of the patient's general health status. It is true that the roentgenogram of the chest will reveal the presence of coarctation of the aorta, but this diagnosis should be made on physical examination rather than on roentgenogram of the chest.

Urinary catecholamines and/or metabolites   The indications for performing tests to rule out phaeochromocytoma are listed in Table 6. Retrospective analysis indicates that the diagnosis of phaeochromocytoma would seldom be missed if these criteria are observed[15]. When hypertension is sustained, the most reliable screening procedure for phaeochromocytoma is determination of the 24h urinary excretion of

Table 6   Indications for performing tests for phaeochromocytoma

Symptomatic paroxysms of hypertension
Headache, tachycardia, palpitations, tremor
Excessive sweating, paroxysmal or continuous
Hypertensive retinopathy (group III or IV)
Unusual lability of blood pressure
Substandard weight or recent weight loss
Hypermetabolism without hyperthyroidism
Abnormal carbohydrate metabolism
Short history of hypertension (< 2 years)
Pressor response to antipressor drugs or during induction of anaesthesia

metanephrines[16]. Determinations of urinary VMA or free catecholamines have been less reliable than the metanephrines. When hypertension is intermittent, indicating that the tumour may not be functioning continuously a provocative test using either histamine or glucagon intravenously should be performed immediately before starting a 24-h collection of urine for metanephrines, to be certain that the tumour has been stimulated to secrete catecholamine.

Peripheral venous renin activity (PVRA)   In spite of the fact that several authors have recommended that peripheral venous renin activity be included as a standard procedure in the routine work-up of the hypertensive patient[17–20], it is not recommended by the ICHD report[9], the report of the Joint National Committee[10] or by other authors[21–23]. The PVRA has not been a reliable screening test for renovascular hypertension and most patients with suppressed PVRA do not have primary aldosteronism. PVRA must always be related to sodium balance, which is difficult in the ambulatory patient. Previous suggestions that PVRA has prognostic and therapeutic implications have not been confirmed[21–23].

Adrenal corticosteroids   Determinations of plasma-free cortisol or urinary 17-hydroxycorticoids or 17-ketosteroids, as well as the decadron suppression test, are necessary only when there are clues to the presence of Cushing's syndrome on physical examination described previously.

Urinary and/or plasma aldosterone levels are unnecessary unless unprovoked hypokalaemia with inappropriate kaliuresis has been confirmed.

ECONOMIC CONSIDERATIONS

It is obvious that an elaborate diagnostic evaluation of all 23 million hypertensive patients in the United States, and a similar percentage in some other parts of the world, would have a major economic impact. It has been estimated that the cost of finding a patient with renovascular disease in the United States varies from $2000 to $4000 depending on whether the intravenous pyelogram, the isotope renogram or both are employed for screening[24]. The cost of accomplishing one surgical cure ranges from $14 000 to $20 000. Projecting these figures to the total American hypertensive population, it was calculated that it would cost at least 13 *billion* US dollars to identify and cure an estimated 800 000 patients with renovascular hypertension. This is over 10% of the gross national product allocated for medical resources.

Fortunately, economic considerations are not the major reason for advocating a simplified and streamlined approach to the evaluation of the hypertensive patient. The minimal work-up advocated here will accomplish the objectives outlined, making a more elaborate evaluation unnecessary.

SUMMARY

A simplified diagnostic approach to the hypertensive patient is economical, is not so formidable that it will be a deterrent to the physician or the patient and will accomplish the objectives that are sought. Subsequently, if the hypertension does not respond adequately to medical treatment, or the patient does not cooperate with the medical regimen, a more elaborate and extensive investigation is indicated to be certain that a potentially curable cause has not been overlooked.

References

1 Tucker, R. M. and Labarthe, D. R. (1977). Frequency of surgical treatment at the Mayo Clinic from 1973 through 1975. *Mayo Clin. Proc.*, **52**, 549

2 Gifford, R. W., Jr (1963). Evaluation of the hypertensive patient with emphasis on detecting curable causes. *Milbank Mem. Fund Q.*, **37**, 170

3 Veterans Administration Cooperative Study Group on Antihypertensive Agents. (1967). *Effects of Treatment on Morbidity in Hypertension*. I. Results in Patients with diastolic blood pressure averaging 115 through 129 mmHg. *J. Amer. Med. Assoc.*, **202**, 1028

4 Veterans Administration Cooperative Study Group on Antihypertensive Agents. (1970). *Effects of Treatment on Morbidity in Hypertension*. II. Results in patients with diastolic blood pressure averaging 90 through 114 mmHg. *J. Amer. Med. Assoc.*, **213**, 1143

5 Gifford, R. W., Jr (1973). Evaluation of the hypertensive patient. *Chest*, **64**, 336

6 Moser, M. (1973). A simplified approach to hypertension. *Am. Fam. Physician*, **7**, 117

7 Wilber, J. A. (1977). The minimum work-up for hypertension. *Cardiovasc. Med.*, (Jan) pp 55–64

8 Finnerty, F. A., Jr (1975). Extensive hypertensive work-up: Con. *J. Amer Med. Assoc.*, **231**, 402

9 Report of Inter-Society Commission for Heart Disease Resources. (1971). Guidelines for the detection, diagnosis, and management of hypertensive populations. *Circulation*, **44A**, 263

10 Report of the Joint National Committee on detection, evaluation, and treatment of high blood pressure. (1977). A Cooperative Study. *J. Amer. Med. Assoc.*, **237**, 255

11 Breslin, D. J., Gifford, R. W., Jr, Fairbairn, J. F., II and Kearns, T. P. (1966). Prognostic importance of ophthalmoscopic findings in essential hypertension. *J. Amer. Med. Assoc.*, **195**, 335

12 Tarazi, R. C., Frohlich, E. D., Dustan, H. P., Gifford, R. W., Jr. and Page, I. H. (1966). Hypertension and high hematocrit. Another clue to renal arterial disease. *Am. J. Cardiol.*, **18**, 855

13 Bookstein, J. J., Abrams, H. L., Buenger, R. D., Lecky, J., Franklin, S. S., Reiss, M.D., Bleifer, K. H., Klatte, E. C., Varady, P. D. and Maxwell, M. H. (1972). Co-operative Study of Renovascular Hypertension. *Radiologic Aspects of Renovascular Hypertension*. Part 2. The role of urography unilateral renovascular disease. *J. Amer. Med. Assoc.*, **220**, 1225

14 Hughes, J. S., Dove, H. S., Gifford, R. W., Jr and Feinstein, A. R. (1977). Non-invasive predictors of surgical cure for renovascular hypertension. (Abst). *Clin. Research*, **25**, 442A

15 Gifford, R. W., Jr, Kvale, W. F., Maher, F. T., Roth, G. M. and Priestley, J. T. (1964). Clinical features, diagnosis and treatment of pheochromocytoma: A review of 76 cases. *Mayo Clin. Proc.*, **39**, 281

16 DeOreo, G. A., Jr, Stewart, B. H., Tarazi, R. C. and Gifford, R. W., Jr (1974). Blood transfusion in the safe surgical management of pheochromocytoma: A review of 46 cases. *J. Urology*, **111**, 715

17 Grim, C. E., Weinberger, M. H., Higgins, J. T. and Kramer, N. J. (1977). Diagnosis of secondary forms of hypertension. *J. Amer. Med. Assoc.*, **237**, 1331

18 Wallach, L., Nyarai, I. and Dawson, K. G. (1975). Stimulated renin: A screening test for hypertension. *Ann. Intern. Med.*, **82**, 27

19 Bühler, F. R., Laragh, J. H., Baer, L., Vaughan, E. D. and Brunner, H. R. (1972). Propranolol inhibition of renin secretion. *N. Engl. J. Med.*, **287**, 1209

20 Brunner, H. R., Laragh, J. H., Baer, L., Newton, M. A., Goodwin, F. T., Krakoff, L. R., Bard, R. H. and Bühler, F. R. (1972). Essential hypertension: renin and aldosterone, heart attack and stroke. *N. Engl. J. Med.*, **286**, 441

21 Kaplan, N. M. (1977). Renin profiles. *J. Amer. Med. Assoc.*, **238**, 611

22 Kaplan, N. M. (1975). The prognostic implications of plasma renin in essential hypertension. *J. Amer. Med Assoc.*, **231**, 167

23 Gifford, R. W. Jr (1977). Renin and the evaluation of the hypertensive patient. *Practical Cardiology* (Aug), pp 55–56

24 McNeil, B. J., Varady, P. D., Burrows, B. A. and Adelstein, S. J. (1975). Measures of clinical efficacy. Cost-effectiveness calculations in the diagnosis and treatment of hypertensive renovascular disease. *N. Engl. J. Med.*, **293**, 216

4

Haemodynamic effects of antihypertensive agents

P. Lund-Johansen

INTRODUCTION: HAEMODYNAMIC ALTERATIONS IN HYPER-
TENSION

In most patients with hypertension the cause is unknown and so are most
of the mechanisms initiating and maintaining the elevated blood
pressure. If these mechanisms were fully understood and were correctable by drugs, a truly rational therapy would be possible.

One approach is to identify the major haemodynamic disturbances
and correct these by drugs. Such therapy would seem to be a logical approach even if the exact mechanisms behind the corrections were not
fully understood.

The arterial blood pressure (BP) may be raised by an increase in the
cardiac output (CO) or in the total peripheral resistance (TPR) or in
both these factors according to the following equation:

$$MAP = CO \times TPR \quad \text{or} \quad MAP = (HR \times SV) \times TPR$$

(MAP = mean arterial pressure, SV = stroke volume, HR = heart
rate)[1]. The CO and TPR may be changed by functional or structural
alterations directly in the heart or in the resistance vessels, or via changes
in their sympathetic or parasympathetic tone, by changes in the plasma
volume or in the capacitance vessels.

The haemodynamic pattern differs greatly from patient to patient,
depending on the type of hypertension, the degree of pressure elevation
and the stage of the hypertensive process. In *essential* hypertension it is
well documented that in young subjects without complications (WHO
stage I) the CO at rest is higher than in normotensive age-matched controls while the calculated TPR is not elevated. The high CO is associated
with an increase in HR and in body oxygen consumption, the cause of

61

which is unknown. During exercise, the CO is no longer increased, but subnormal (due to insufficient increase in SV) and the TPR does not fall to the same low levels as in normotensive subjects[2].

In subjects with established hypertension, but without target organ complications (WHO stage I–II), the CO at rest is normal or subnormal; during exercise it is clearly reduced and the oxygen delivery to the tissues is provided by an increase in the arteriovenous oxygen difference. The TPR is increased at rest as well as during exercise.

In subjects with hypertension and cardiovascular complications (WHO stage III), the CO and SV are markedly reduced at rest as well as during exercise, and the TPR is greatly increased, disturbances probably reflecting pronounced structural changes in the left ventricle and in the resistance vessels[3]. Figure 1 summarizes these findings.

Thus the circulatory system will usually be very different in a young man in WHO stage I compared with an old man in stage II or III. With the same arterial pressure, the resistance in the older man might be twice that in the younger, and the blood flow (CO) only half. The tolerance to drug-induced reduction in CO in these two situations might be very different.

Recent long-term studies in subjects with untreated essential hypertension have shown that the CO drops and the TPR increases over the years, more than expected by normal ageing[4]. These changes possibly reflect a gradual restructuring of the high-pressure compartments in hypertension, according to Folkow's concept[5].

Studies of the *regional* circulation have demonstrated that the resistance seems to be increased in most vascular areas, most in the kidneys and in the splanchnic and cutaneous circulation[6].

The haemodynamic changes in *secondary* hypertension (found in about 5% of an unselected hypertensive population) will not be discussed here. In most forms TPR is increased as in essential hypertension[7]. In patients with hypertension and severe renal failure changes in plasma volume are of particular importance for regulation of the CO and the BP[8].

It is beyond the scope of this chapter to discuss the disturbances in the control mechanisms responsible for the changes in the central haemodynamics. An excellent overview has recently been published by Birkenhäger and Schalekamp[9].

THE ANTIHYPERTENSIVE AGENTS

The antihypertensive agents can be classified under three main categories: (1) diuretics; (2) drugs acting on the nervous system; and (3)

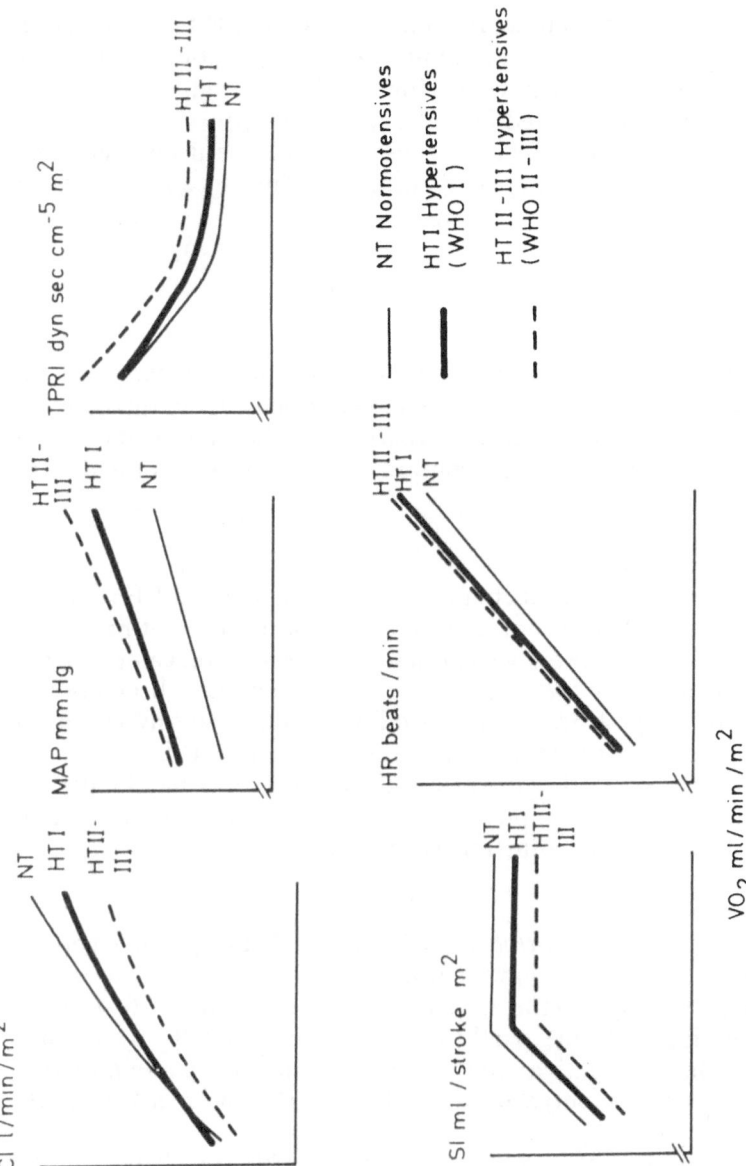

Figure 1 Diagram of central haemodynamics in normotensives and hypertensives at rest and during exercise. VO₂ = oxygen consumption, CI = cardiac index, MAP = mean arterial pressure, TPRI = total peripheral resistance index, SI = stroke index, HR = heart rate. Note the change in haemodynamic pattern in transition from rest to exercise in the hypertensive group in WHO stage I. Also note the difference between this group and patients in stage II or III

vasodilators.

Each of these main groups will initially lower the blood pressure by very different mechanisms – such as reduction in CO via increased diuresis and fall in plasma volume; reduction in CO or TPR via changes in nervous tone to the heart or resistance vessels; reduction in TPR via direct affect on the arteriolar wall. However, the initial effects may be obscured or even counteracted by reflexogenic compensatory reactions. To complicate the study of the antihypertensive mechanisms even more, long-term pressure reduction, *per se*, seems to induce secondary changes in CO and TPR.

DIURETICS

In most patients with hypertension there is no obvious excess of salt and water in the body; nevertheless removal of NaCl from the body has been an important principle in antihypertensive therapy for more than 50 years. The *Kempner rich diet*, containing about 200 mg of NaCl, is a well-known example.

The mercurial diuretics

The mercurial diuretics, used about 25 years ago, lowered BP in hypertensive patients, but were not suitable for long-term treatment. The great breakthrough in the drug treatment of hypertension came in 1957, with the discovery of the *thiazide diuretics*. They have now been used for 20 years as the drug of first choice in mild and moderate hypertension and as a supplement to other drugs in more severe forms[10].

The diuretics used in therapy of hypertension today may be divided into three groups: thiazides and similar compounds; short-acting, highly potent loop diuretics; and potassium sparing diuretics.

The thiazide diuretics

The first thiazide was *chlorothiazide* with relatively low potency per mg, the common daily dose being in the order of 1000 mg. Later *hydrochlorothiazide* was developed – the usual daily dose being about 50–100 mg. By changing this molecule partly by substituting the R_6 by Cl or F (Figure 2), other derivatives like *trichlormethiazide, methylchlothiazide, cyclopenthiazide, polythiazide* and *bendroflumethiazide* were developed[11]

The thiazide diuretics block the reabsorption of Na and Cl in the distal tubules. Potassium excretion is also increased. In hypertensive patients continuous administration leads to the so-called 'escape phenomenon' – the excretion of Na and Cl stabilizes, and an equilibrium is obtained[12].

The various thiazides lower BP through the same mechanism, and they are equal regarding BP-lowering effect, although their dose and duration of effects vary.

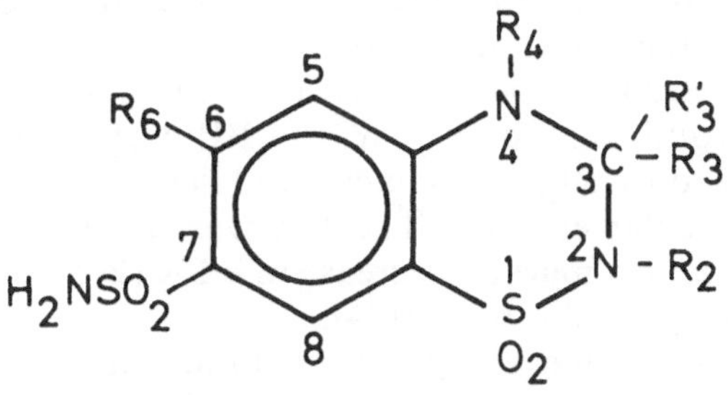

Figure 2 The thiazide molecule

Absorption and excretion The thiazides are rapidly absorbed from the gastrointestinal tract, and show a high degree of plasma-binding. The thiazides are excreted in the proximal tubule, but partly reabsorbed again. Most derivatives are excreted within 3–6 h, polythiazide is considerably slower. After an oral dose the diuretic effect is apparent after 2–4 h, with maximal effect after 6–8 h. Total duration is about 12–24 h (polythiazide 24–48 h),[11,13].

The dose–response curve is relatively flat. If the dose is increased above the common therapeutic level very little additional BP reduction is achieved.

Haemodynamic effects
Acute and semi-acute effects Intravenous injection of 500–1000 mg chlorothiazide in hypertensive patients induce a rapid drop in CO due to reduction in SV with no change in HR. TPR increases and BP is unchanged or only slightly reduced[14–17].

When the thiazides are given orally over several days, the BP falls, because the compensatory increase in TPR disappears; the TPR falls to pre-treatment levels or slightly lower. However, the CO remains reduced because of a persistent decrease in SV, and HR remains unchanged. The increased diuresis during several days causes a reduction in the plasma volume of about 10–15% with a fall in venous return[18–20].

However, this effect alone cannot explain the antihypertensive effect of the thiazides, because when the plasma volume is raised to pre-treatment level by infusions of dextran the blood pressure will not always rise[21,22]. In this phase it has been shown that there is a reduced pressure response to catecholamines, possibly due to the hypovolaemia[23].

Long-term effects   In 1960 Conway and Lauwers reported that chloro-thiazide given to patients with hypertension over a period of several months resulted in a decrease in BP, a gradual increase in CO to pre-treatment level and a fall in TPR – in other words a change towards normal in central haemodynamics[20].

In a personal study in patients with essential hypertension treated with hydrochlorothiazide for 1 year, the BP dropped significantly. At rest the CO was only slightly reduced and remained at pre-treatment level during muscular exercise. The HR was unchanged, and the BP reduction was due to a marked decrease in TPR (Figure 3)[24]. A study of polythiazide gave similar results[24].

Our study showed that the plasma volume was 240 ml lower than before treatment. Other recent studies[25,26] have also demonstrated this persistent reduction in plasma volume which was first reported by Wilson and Freis in 1959[27].

As a consequence of the plasma volume decrease, plasma renin is increased[28].

It is still uncertain how the TPR is decreased by long-term treatment with thiazides. Extensive reviews of the various theories have been presented by Tarazi[29] and by Freis[30].

Chlorthalidone

Chlorthalidone differs from most thiazides in having a longer effect – 24–48 h. Dose-range is 25–50 mg every day or 50–100 mg every second day[11].

A daily dose of 200 mg chlorthalidone for about 10 days given to hypertensive patients induced a reduction in BP associated with a decrease in CO and no change in TPR, exactly like the thiazides[31].

Mefruside

The diuretic effect of mefruside is rather similar to that of the thiazide diuretics. The maximal effect is seen after 6–10 h. The antihypertensive mode of action is probably the same[32].

Side-effects of thiazides and similar agents

The most important side-effects of thiazides, chlorthalidone and mefru-side are hypokalaemia, hyperuricaemia, and a diabetogenic effect. The hypokalaemia and hyperuricaemia are directly related to the renal effects of the drugs – increased excretion of K and decreased excretion of uric acid. The increased blood glucose level is possibly due to increased glycogenolysis in the liver and the muscles[10–12,33]

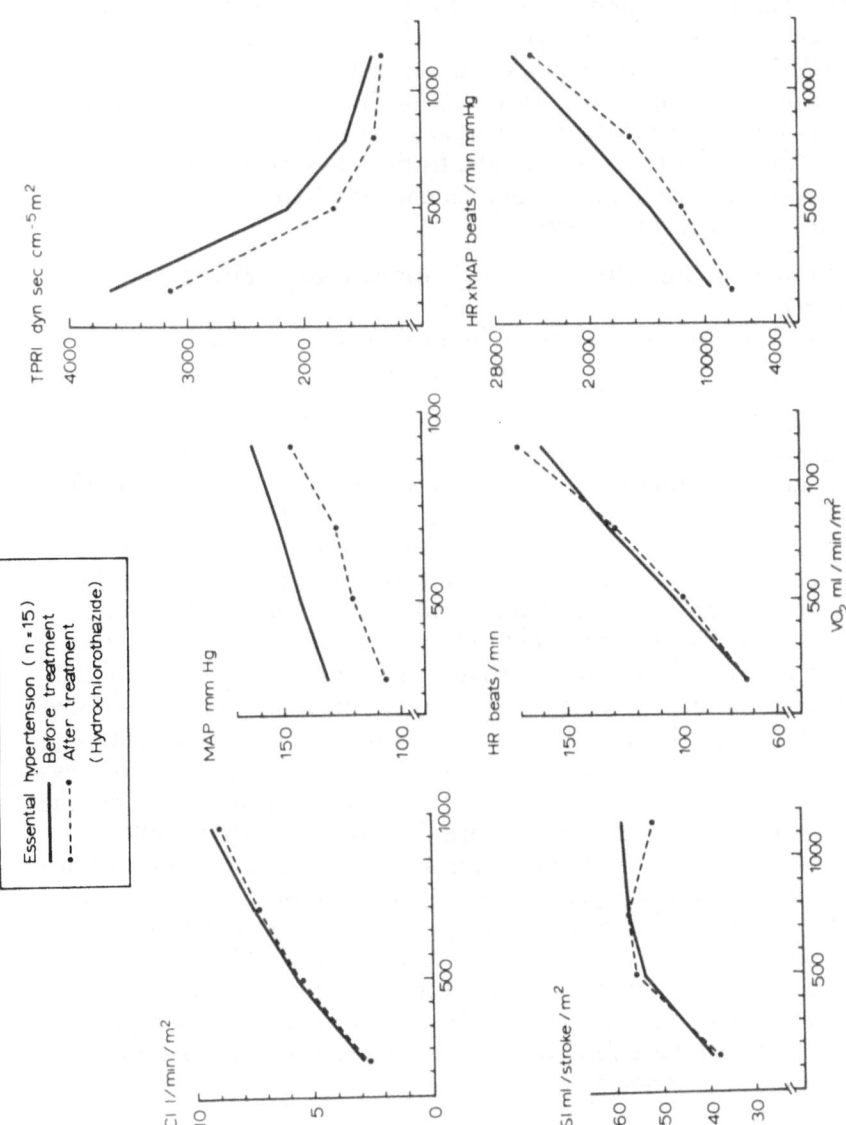

Figure 3 Haemodynamic alterations induced by 1-year treatment with hydrochlorothiazide. Legend as in Figure 1. Note the marked decrease in TPRI at rest as well as during exercise, and the unchanged HR. Also note the relatively small effect on pressure–heart rate product

Short-acting highly potent loop diuretics (furosemide, ethacrynic acid, bumetanid)

It is well documented that the short-acting, highly potent diuretics furosemide, etacrynic acid and bumetanid also lower the BP[10,34,35], and the haemodynamic effects are thought to be the same as for the thiazide diuretics[35]. However, as a marked diuresis during the first hours after an oral dose is common and disturbing to the patients, and since their duration of action is rather short, these drugs are not recommended for use in ordinary hypertensive patients. In situations such as hypertensive crisis, hypertension and pulmonary oedema and hypertension and renal failure these drugs are very useful.

Potassium-sparing diuretics (spironolactone, triamterene and amilorid)

Only spironolactone is used alone in antihypertensive therapy, and the two other agents will not be discussed, although they sometimes are useful as supplements to thiazides.

Spironolactone

Spironolactone inhibits the action of aldosterone in distal tubules, induces increased excretion of NaCl and water and reduction in potassium excretion. It is indicated in patients with primary aldosteronism, permanently or prior to surgical therapy[36]. Overproduction of aldosterone is uncommon in patients with essential hypertension[9], but spironolactone lowers BP also in most of these patients[37]. Some authors have reported a particularly good response in patients with high plasma volume and low plasma renin activity[38]; others have found the antihypertensive effect to be independent of these factors[37]. In a recent long-term study in patients with essential hypertension the BP drop was mainly due to decreased TPR (at rest). During exercise, however, the reduction in BP was related to decreases in both CO and TPR[39].

The solubility and absorption of spironolactone in the intestine is critically dependent on the particle size. The 'micronized' form is best absorbed[11]. Dose-range is 25–50 mg once or twice daily; in patients with primary or secondary aldosteronism it is considerably more[36].

Hyperkalaemia is often seen if the renal function is reduced. This is directly related to spironolactone's effect on the kidneys. In male patients gynaecomastia has been reported. Its mechanism is related to the steroid-like molecule of spironolactone.

DRUGS ACTING ON THE NERVOUS SYSTEM

In the early phase of essential hypertension there is possibly an overactivity of the sympathetic nervous system reflected in increased plasma catecholamines[9]. Apart from this, no definite abnormalities in the nervous system have been demonstrated in hypertension of various types. Nevertheless, drugs interfering with the *nervous control* of the heart and the blood vessels have been used in therapy of hypertension for about 30 years.

These agents may act at various sites, including centrally in the hypothalamus or vasomotor centre, in the sympathetic and parasympathetic ganglia, in the peripheral sympathetic nerve endings, or in the peripheral adrenergic receptors (alpha- and beta-receptors). Some agents act both centrally and peripherally (Figure 4). They all disturb the metabolism or

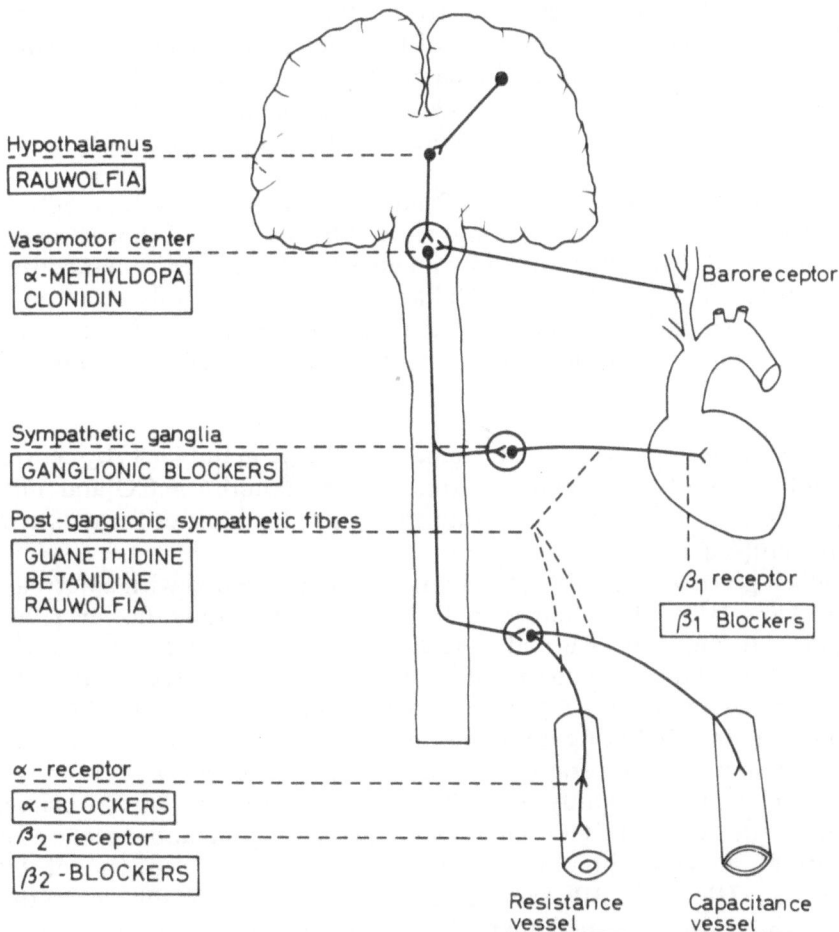

Figure 4 Diagram of site of action of antihypertensive agents acting on the nervous system

storage of noradrenalin, or interfere with receptors normally stimulated by noradrenalin[40–42].

Mainly centrally acting agents

Alpha-methyldopa
Several theories have been advanced to explain the BP-lowering effect of alpha-methyldopa. The present concept is that alpha-methyldopa has a direct action on the lower brain stem, within or near the vasomotor centre. In this area there are BP-modulating centres with alpha-adrenergic receptors. Stimulation of these lead paradoxically to reduction in the BP. Alpha-methyldopa readily penetrates the blood–brain barrier and is metabolized to methyl-noradrenalin. This metabolite stimulates alpha-adrenergic receptors to induce BP reduction[42].

Absorption, excretion   After oral administration only about 50% is absorbed from the gastrointestinal tract. The majority of that absorbed is conjugated in the liver, and only about 10% of the dose is metabolized to alpha-methyl-noradrenalin. Alpha-methyldopa is mainly excreted in the urine. In patients with reduced renal function, excretion is much slower and accumulation occurs. Smaller doses than usual should then be used[41,43].

Haemodynamic effects   Since alpha-methyldopa mainly acts by central modulation in the vasomotor centre, changes in both the CO and TPR might be expected. The dominating effect appears to differ from patient to patient[42].

When given *acutely*, the BP drop is usually associated with a decrease in CO and HR and no change in TPR[44,45]. One study, however, has reported decrease in TPR and no change in CO[46]. The decrease in CO and HR is relatively modest, and is far less than that seen with beta-blockers. Of importance is that renal blood flow is not decreased[47].

During upright tilting an orthostatic BP drop is seen, but in clinical use symptomatic orthostatic hypotension is uncommon[47].

In a long-term study of BP reduction at rest was associated with a decrease in CO and HR and no significant decrease in TPR[48]. During submaximal muscular exercise the effects of the drug on HR and BP were considerably less, probably reflecting that the centrally mediated effects of alpha-methyldopa can be overridden by other regulatory mechanisms in this situation (Figure 5).

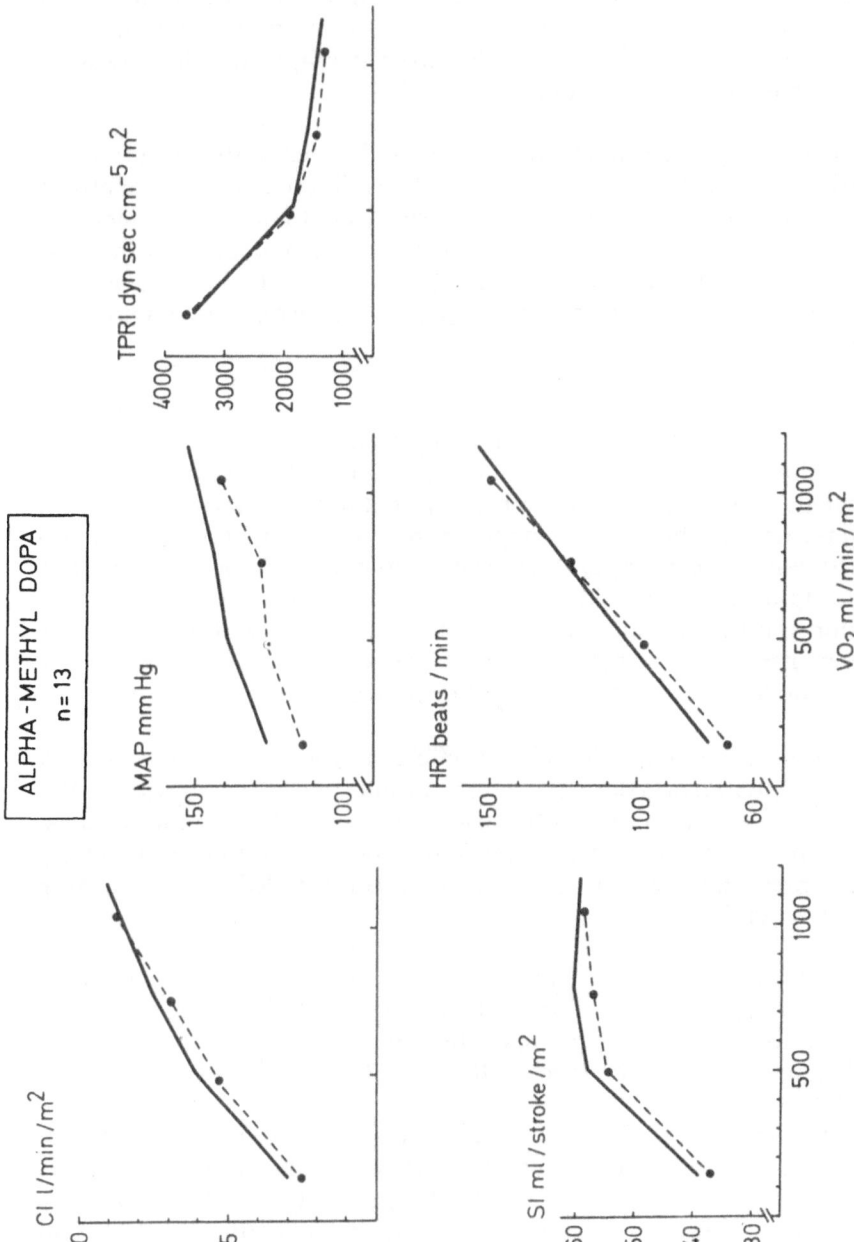

Figure 5 Haemodynamic alterations induced by 1-year treatment with alpha-methyldopa. Legend as in Figure 1. (From Ref. 48 with kind permission from *Acta Medica Scandinavica*).

Side-effects   The most common is sedation and lack of initiative, probably caused by depletion of noradrenalin from the brain[42,49]. Alpha-methyldopa might induce a febrile reaction, haemolytic anaemia, positive Coombs test and also liver damage, which is possibly due to some sort of autoimmune reaction[50].

Rational use   Since renal blood flow is not decreased, the drug is useful in patients with reduced renal function. The reduction in CO is relatively modest and the drug would seem to be safe in patients with moderately reduced CO. Pronounced bradycardia is very uncommon, and the drug has no effect on the bronchioles. It might therefore be used in patients with relatively slow HR and obstructive pulmonary diseases (where beta-blockers are contraindicated).

Clonidine

The mode of action of clonidine is complex but has several similarities with alpha-methyldopa. It stimulates the alpha-adrenergic receptors in or near the vasomotor centre. When injected in the cisterna magna, the result is a drop in the BP via changes in the sympathetic tone of the heart and the resistance vessels[51]. However, clonidine also acts peripherally on the alpha-receptors in the resistance vessels where it causes vasoconstriction. Thus, when clonidine is injected peripherally, it has a biphasic BP response: first a rise due to peripheral vasoconstriction, and then a drop as the centrally mediated effect begins to dominate[52] (Figure 6).

Absorption, excretion   Clonidine is effective when given intravenously or orally. After an oral dose maximum plasma concentration is seen after about 2 h [53]. Plasma half life varies from 6 to 23 h. Clonidine is extremely potent per mg, the ordinary oral dose is around 200–600 μg daily. Intravenously 100–200 g is recommended as a starting dose (injected slowly!).

Haemodynamic effects   Acute injection of 150–300 μg clonidine intravenously results in a rise of BP of about 15% lasting a few minutes, folowed by a prolonged fall in the BP associated with a significant decrease in the HR and CO and no change in TPR[52]

Haemodynamic changes seen after 1 week on oral therapy are identical with the acute changes[54]. In a 1 year study in patients with essential hypertension 300–600 μg daily induced a 16% reduction in BP at rest associated with a reduction in HR and CO and only slight decrease in TPR[52]. During muscular exercise the effect on the BP was modest, similar to that seen

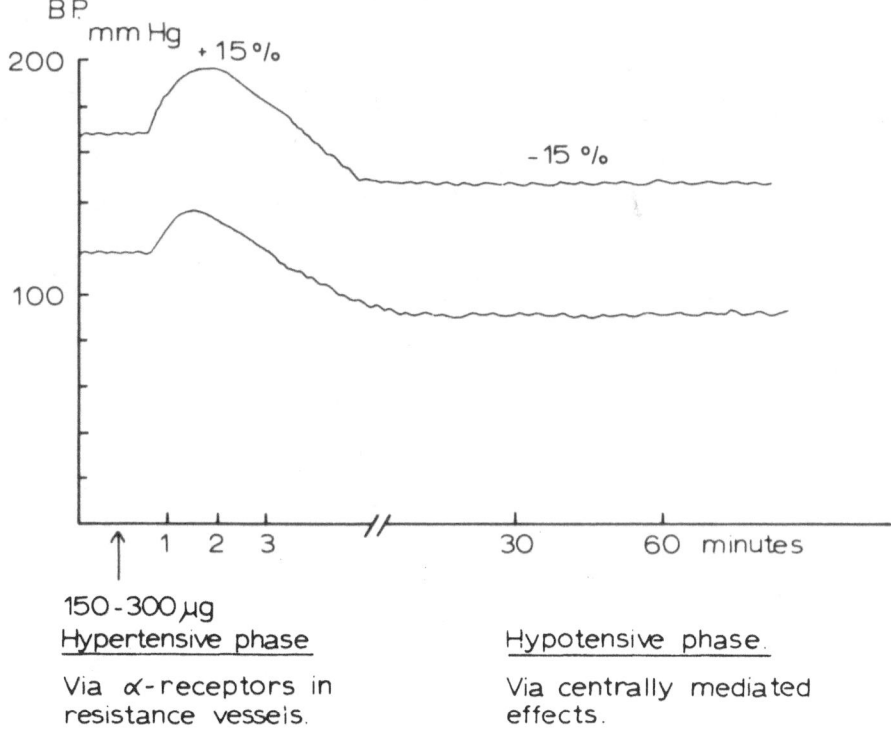

Figure 6 Blood pressure response after injection of clonidine peripherally. Note the immediate hypertensive phase followed by a prolonged hypotensive phase

during long-term therapy with alpha-methyldopa (Figure 7).

Side-effects and rational use Like alpha-methyldopa clonidine frequently causes sedation and dry mouth. Clonidine does not seem to induce haemolytic anaemia, positive Coombs test or liver damage. However, a drawback with clonidine is a risk of hypertensive crisis if the drug is withdrawn suddenly[55].

Clonidine seems to have haemodynamic effects resembling those of alpha-methyldopa, and may be used for the same indications.

Ganglionic blockers
The ganglionic blockers now belong to history. Great disturbances in the orthostatic BP control and frequent side-effects from other organs have made the ganglionic blockers obsolete for the therapy of hypertension[41].

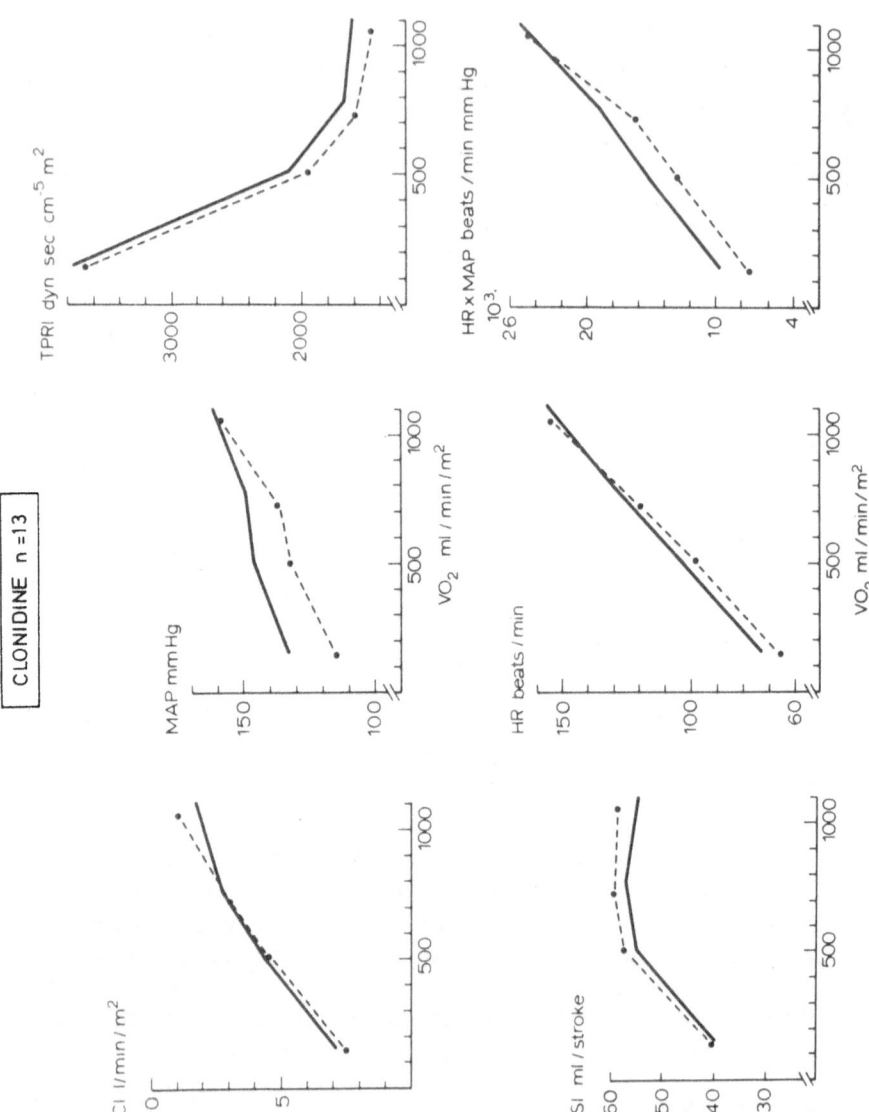

Figure 7 Haemodynamic changes induced by 1-year treatment with clonidine. Note the modest effect on HR and MAP during severe muscular exercise

Mainly peripherally acting agents

Guanethidine and betanidine
Guanethidine and betanidine are post-ganglionic adrenolytic drugs. They act exclusively on the peripheral sympathetic nervous system where they interfere with the normal metabolism of noradrenalin. The two agents have very similar actions, but betanidine acts much more rapidly and for a shorter period than guanethidine. Betanidine given orally will lower BP within a few hours, while it might take days to reduce BP with guanethidine[41,56,57].

Both drugs reduce BP by interfering with the sympathetic tone to the heart, resistance vessels and the capacitance vessels. In acute studies the effect on the capacitance vessels appears first, and is often very marked. The CO is markedly reduced. Orthostatic BP drop is often very pronounced[58,59].

Agents with both central and peripheral effect

Rauwolfia alkaloids
The rauwolfia alkaloids deplete the central and peripheral stores of noradrenalin in the nerve terminals. The effect, however, is cumulative and lasts several weeks. As an important side-effect of rauwolfia alkaloids is mental depression, sometimes ending in suicide, this cumulative and long-lasting effect is undesirable.

Acute injection of 2–3 mg reserpine intravenously will usually induce a reduction in the TPR, in some patients also a reduction in CO associated with bradycardia. A slight reduction in glomerular filtration rate has been noted[60].

In long-term studies reduction in the TPR and no great changes in the CO have been reported[61].

Although the rauwolfia alkaloids seem to have a favourable haemodynamic reaction pattern, their side-effects make them less desirable than other agents available today. In many countries they are not used in long term therapy any more.

Adrenergic receptor blocking agents

Beta-adrenoceptor blocking agents (beta-blockers)
The beta-blocker propranolol was introduced in therapy of hypertension in 1964 by Prichard[62]. These drugs interfere with the sympathetic control of the heart by blocking the beta$_1$-receptors in the heart and the beta$_2$-receptors which control bronchial dilatation, dilatation of blood vessels in striated muscle only and several other functions. For the sake

of simplicity drugs acting predominantly on the beta$_1$-receptors are termed *cardioselective*. Agents blocking both the cardiac beta$_1$-receptors and the beta$_2$-receptors are termed *non-cardioselective*. Some beta-blockers also have a stimulating effect on the receptors, the so-called intrinsic sympathicomimetic activity (ISA).

All types of beta-blockers, whether cardioselective, non-cardioselective, with or without ISA, are able to reduce BP in the majority of patients with essential hypertension and in a large fraction of patients with secondary hypertension. It is beyond the scope of this chapter to discuss the various theories which try to explain why BP is reduced by beta-blockers. Recent reviews have been published by Birkenhäger *et al.*[63] and Tarazi[64].

Absorption excretion   The beta-blockers are easily absorbed from the gastrointestinal tract. The bioavailability differs mainly due to differences in the first pass elimination in the liver[65]. The beta-blockers and their metabolites are excreted in the urine.

Haemodynamic effects

(i) Non-cardioselective beta-blockers without ISA. When 10–15 mg of *propranolol* are given intravenously to hypertensive patients, the CO falls due to a marked decrease in HR and a small reduction in SV. The TPR rises and the BP is unchanged. A similar reaction pattern is seen with *timolol*[66–71].

During long-term treatment with propranolol the TPR falls, the CO and the HR remains reduced and the BP drops[64,67,72,73].

During muscular exercise the BP is reduced compared to pre-treatment level and there is a substantial decrease in HR and CO[74]. The TPR stays at pre-treatment level or is slightly increased. There is a substantial reduction in the pressure heart rate product of about 40% at rest as well as during exercise. Timolol induces a similar reaction pattern[75,76] (Figure 8).

(ii) Other beta-blockers.   The non-cardioselective beta-blockers with ISA like alprenolol[66,77] and pindolol[78] and the cardioselective beta-blockers like atenolol[79,80] and metoprolol[81] seem to reduce BP largely through the same mechanisms as propranolol. Some differences seem to exist with respect to the SV and TPR responses, but since it is uncertain whether these differences are of any clinical importance, they will not be discussed here. The haemodynamic long-term effect of atenolol[80] is shown in Figure 9.

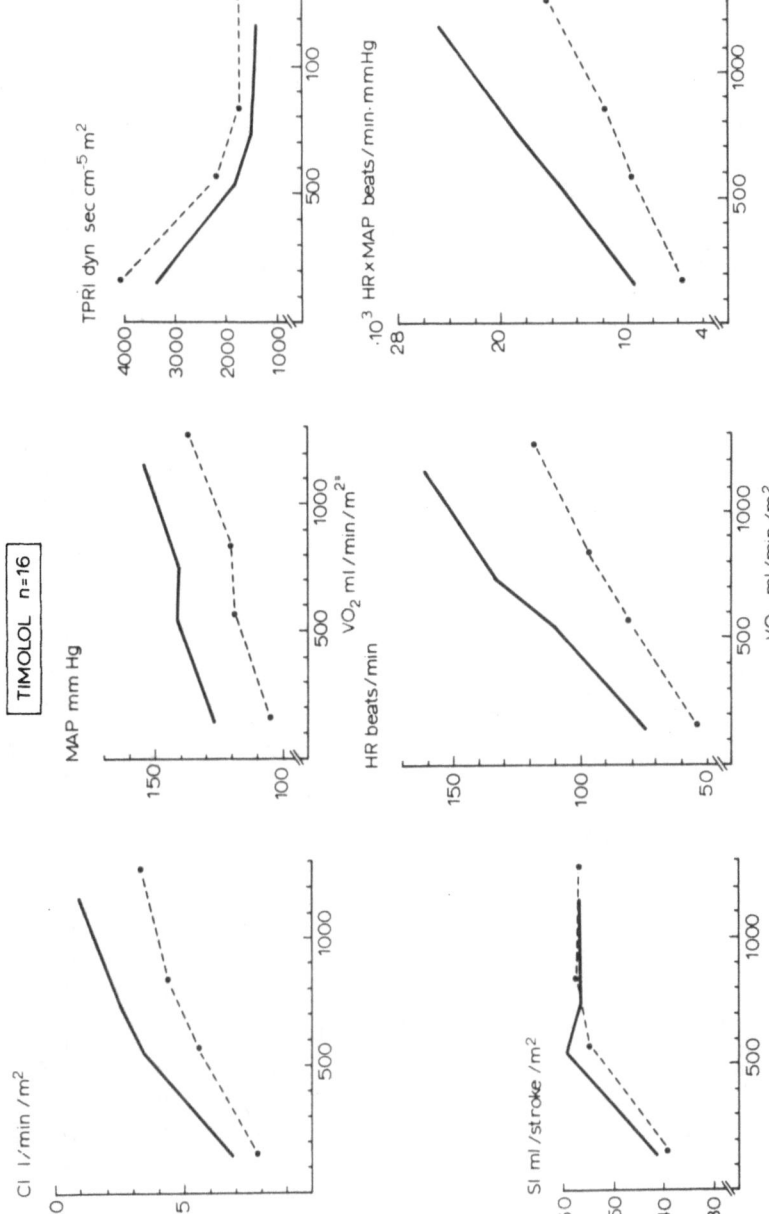

Figure 8 Haemodynamic changes induced by 1-year treatment with timolol. Note the dramatic decrease in HR and in HR–MAP product. Legend as in Figure 1. (From Ref. 75 with kind permission from *Acta Medica Scandinavica*)

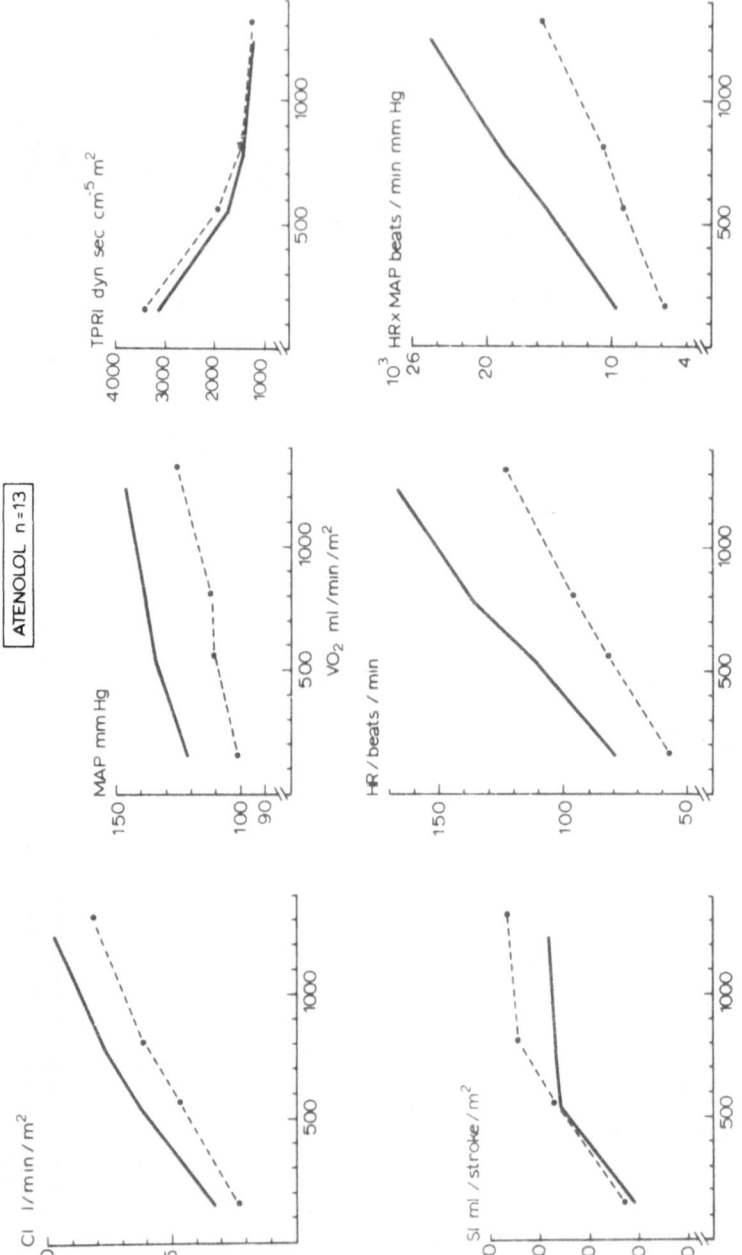

Figure 9 Haemodynamic changes induced by 1-year treatment with atenolol. Note the differences from timolol (Figure 8) with respect to TPRI and SI. Legend as in Figure 1. (From Ref. 80 with kind permission from *British Journal of Clinical Pharmacology*)

Side-effects   Blockade of the beta$_1$-receptors in the heart might precipitate or worsen heart failure, bradycardia and A-V block. Blockade of the beta$_2$-receptors in the bronchioles might increase airway resistance, provoke asthma and reduce or abolish the therapeutic effect of bronchodilators. The reduction in CO will decrease blood flow to several organ systems, and in particular patients with obliterating arterial diseases will often become worse. Thus heart failure (manifest or latent), severe bradycardia, A-V block grade II or III, obliterating arterial disease, chronic bronchitis or asthma should be regarded as *contraindications*. When these are respected, side-effects from beta-blockers are few.

Most beta-blockers pass the blood–brain barrier where they are thought to have effects on the central nervous system. In some patients a slight sedative effect may occur. More important side-effects from the central nervous system are disturbances in sleep, sometimes with nightmares or vivid dreams.

Rational use   Apart from subjects at rest with mild essential hypertension, the beta-blockers do not change central haemodynamics in a favourable direction, particularly not during muscular exercise. BP is reduced at the expense of CO and blood flow to several organ systems. In patients who prior to treatment have a normal or only slightly reduced CO, the reduction in CO seems to be surprisingly well tolerated[77,80,81], although disturbances in liver enzymes, in lactate and pyruvate metabolism in the muscles have been reported[82]. However, most patients are able to perform ordinary physical exercise without any obvious changes in performance. The beta-blockers have several other advantages. The marked reduction in HR and BP results in great reduction in the work-load on the heart and thus the beta-blockers are of particular value in patients with hypertension and angina pectoris. One should also expect that hypertensive patients with high HR and high CO would be particularly suitable for beta-blockade. Most patients who complain of tachycardia, palpitations or cardiac awareness, will become free of these symptoms. However, other patients without elevated CO also respond to the beta-blockers, although it should be remembered that in older patients there is an increased risk of inducing heart failure.

Antiarrhythmic effect   An important cause of death in hypertensive patients is myocardial infarction with ventricular tachycardia or fibrillation. Some studies have demonstrated that the beta-blockers might reduce the risk of such malignant arrhythmias[83,84]. If this is further documented it is possible that the beta-blockers will be used not only for their BP-lowering effect but also to prevent sudden death and fatal myocardial infarction by their antiarrhythmic action.

Alpha-adrenoceptor blocking agents (alpha-blockers)
As TPR is increased in most patients with established hypertension and the resistance vessels are controlled by the alpha-adrenergic receptors, the use of alpha-blockers would seem to be a logical approach to treatment in most forms of hypertension. However, although BP may be reduced by injection of such compounds (like *phentolamine* and *phenoxybenzamine)*, the reflexogenic increase in HR and CO tends to counteract the BP drop. Attempts to use these drugs chronically have not been successful due to gastrointestinal side-effects, severe orthostatic hypotension and refractoriness to the effect[85]. Thus these drugs have no place in the therapy of essential hypertension. However, they are of value pre- and peroperatively in patients with phaeochromocytoma.

When combined with beta-blockers in order to inhibit the reflexogenic increase in HR and CO, alpha-blockers will reduce BP. However, the clinical results have been disappointing[87].

Drugs with alpha – and beta-blocking properties
Labetalol   Labetalol is a new antihypertensive drug with an alpha-blocking effect of about one-tenth of the effect of phentolamine, and a beta-blocking effect of one-quarter of the effect of propranolol[88]. Labetalol is readily absorbed from the gastrointestinal tract. The intravenous dose range is about 50–100 mg, the oral dose range about 200–800 mg daily.

In acute studies the BP is rapidly decreased after a few minutes, associated with a marked decrease in TPR and a moderate decrease in HR and CO[89]. Preliminary long-term results suggest that there is a marked reduction in TPR and a modest reduction in HR and CO[90].

When given intravenously in doses of about 50–100 mg labetalol decreases BP within a few minutes, and the drug may be used in therapy of hypertensive crisis[91]. An advantage is that the drug may the be continued orally. Patients with mild and moderate essential hypertension seem to respond well.

VASODILATORS

Drugs acting directly on the smooth muscle of the arteriolar wall inducing dilatation would seem to be a logical approach to most types of hypertension. Unfortunately the BP drop will be counteracted through a reflex increase in HR and CO. However, if the reflexogenic tachycardia is inhibited by a beta-blocker, a marked BP reduction is often achieved.

If the vasodilator also acts on the capacitance vessels, a reduction in the venous return and CO will be achieved which will contribute to the fall of BP.

Hydralazine
Hydralazine has a direct effect on the *myogenic* tone of the resistance vessels. Since the sympathetic innervation of the resistance and capacitance vessels is not affected there is no orthostatic hypotension[92].

Absorption, excretion   Hydralazine is well absorbed from the gastrointestinal tract. An important route of elimination is via the liver, which acetylates hydralazine to products which are excreted in the urine. This reaction is dependent on the enzyme acetyltransferase. Low activity of this enzyme system (seen in so-called 'slow acetylators') involves risk of overdose and side-effects[95].

Haemodynamic effects
After injection of hydralazine there is an immediate drop in the BP due to a marked decrease in TPR. The HR increases and so does the CO. In the arm there is a marked decrease in the TPR and increase in blood flow[92].

Side-effects and rational use
The most severe side-effect of hydralazine is a syndrome resembling lupus erythematosus disseminatus (LED). The mechanism behind this reaction is unknown, but it is mainly patients who are slow acetylators who carry the risk of this side-effect.

Hydralazine should never be used alone, only together with a beta-blocker or similar drug. As the blood flow to the kidneys increases, the drug is particularly useful in patients with hypertension and decreased renal function[94].

Prazosin
The hypotensive effect of prazosin is due to arteriolar dilatation, probably caused by partial blockade of postsynaptic alpha-adrenergic receptors. The drug prevents the reflexogenic rise in HR which occurs with other vasodilators. Thus, the mode of action clearly differs from that of hydralazine, and prazosin may be used alone[95].

Absorption, excretion   Prazosin is easily absorbed when given orally. It is excreted mainly by the kidneys; the daily dose range is about 3–30mg.

Haemodynamics
Studies of the acute effect in patients with moderate essential hypertension have demonstrated that the BP drop is associated with a marked decrease in the TPR, a slight increase in the CO and no significant changes in the HR[96].

In a study in patients with essential hypertension in WHO stage I given 3–7 mg prazosin daily over a year, the BP drop was associated with a consistent decrease in TPR at rest as well as during exercise. At rest HR and CO were slightly but insignificantly increased as compared to the pre-treatment levels. During exercise the CO was significantly increased[97]. Thus, prazosin corrected the haemodynamic disturbances seen in hypertension (Figure 10).

Side-effects and rational use

The most important side-effects are orthostatic blood pressure drop and syncope, particularly after the *first* dose ('the first dose syncope'). The mechanism is unknown. Somewhat surprisingly, subsequent doses are usually well tolerated.

Prazosin is a relatively new antihypertensive drug and long-term observations are few. From a haemodynamic point of view, the drug is able to correct the most important haemodynamic disturbances in established essential hypertension. The drug is of great value in patients with severe hypertension and reduced renal function since renal blood flow is not reduced. Since the HR is not decreased, the effect on the pressure–heart rate product is small and the drug is less suitable for patients with hypertension and angina.

Diazoxide

Diazoxide has a chemical structure somewhat similar to the thiazide diuretics. However, the drug has no diuretic effect, but rather induces fluid retention. Injected rapidly in doses of 300–600 mg it reduces BP in patients with severe hypertension, and is a useful drug in hypertensive crisis[98].

Haemodynamic studies have shown a drop in BP associated with a fall in the calculated TPR and a simultaneous rise in CO and HR[98,99].

Minoxidil

Minoxidil is also a potent vasodilator reserved for therapy of very severe hypertension resistant to other agents. Haemodynamic studies have shown that the drop in the BP is associated with an increase in the CO and the HR[100]. Unfortunately the drug may induce hypertricosis, which is very disturbing in female patients. Fluid retention is frequent and necessitates the use of a diuretic[28].

DRUG COMBINATIONS

Diuretics and beta-blockers

Several studies have shown a greater BP reduction by combination of these two drugs than by the use of either drug alone. In patients begun on

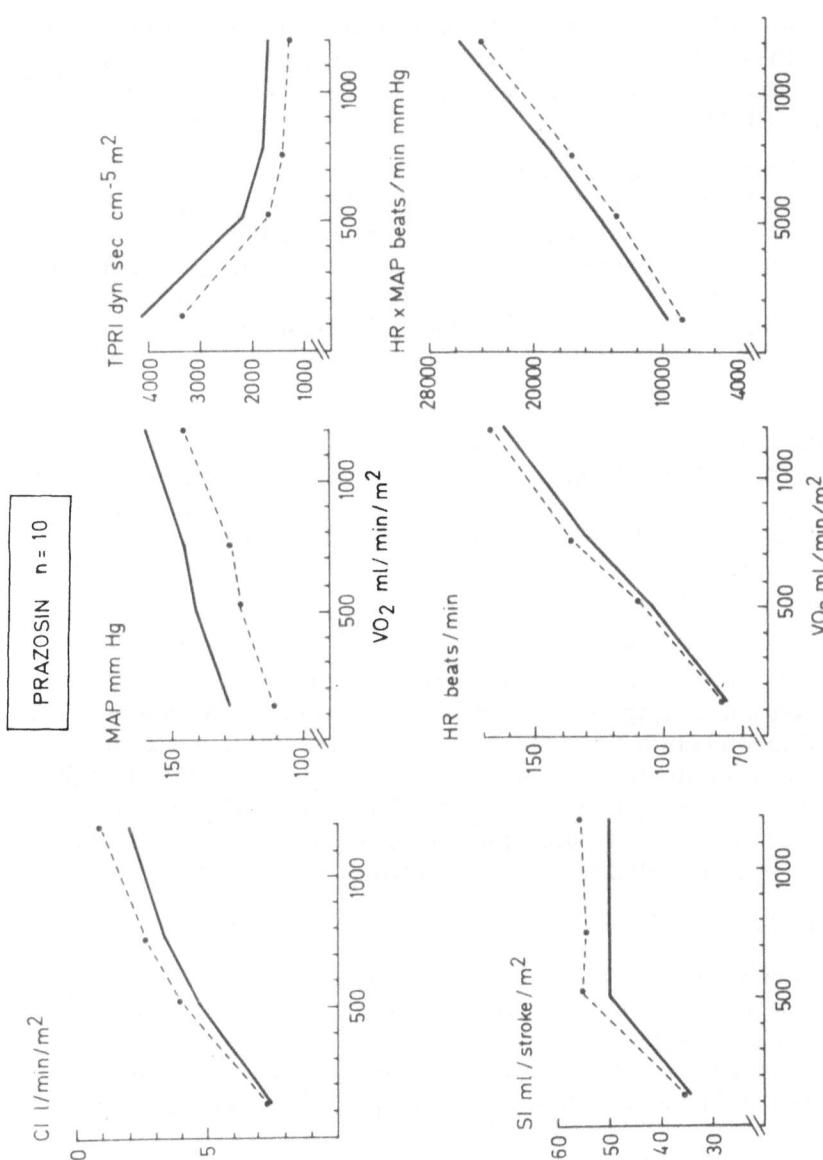

Figure 10 Haemodynamic changes induced by 1-year treatment with prazosin. Note the marked decrease in TPRI and the increase in CI response during muscular exercise. Legend as in Figure 1

a diuretic, the beta-blocker will reduce HR and CO; the TPR, which has been decreased by the thiazide diuretic, will probably remain reduced. Since most beta-blockers lower the renin level, which is raised by the use of diuretics, it has been suggested that this mechanism is partly responsible for the good BP control. However, in many studies there has been no correlation between the decrease in the plasma renin and the reduction in the BP[101].

Sympatholytics and diuretics
In a study of patients treated with sympatholytic drugs with or without diuretics it was found that in patients in whom BP control was satisfactory, the plasma volume was significantly reduced. In patients with unsatisfactory BP reduction, in spite of adequate doses of sympatholytic drugs, plasma volume was relatively high. When diuretic therapy was intensified by furosemide, the plasma volume fell and the BP decreased to satisfactory level[28].

Pure vasodilators and beta-blockers
Hydralazine and beta-blockers have been used extensively in the treatment of moderate and severe hypertension. Acute haemodynamic studies have shown that the reflexogenic rise in HR and CO induced by hydralazine is counteracted by beta-blockers with a resulting greater fall in blood pressure[102, 103].

Prazosin and beta-blockers
In a long-term study of the combination of prazosin and beta-blockers the HR at rest and during exercise was lower than on prazosin alone, but higher than on beta-blockers alone. The SV remained increased and the CO was only slightly reduced during exercise (Figure 11). The BP reduction was greater than on prazosin alone. Thus this combination resulted in a favourable haemodynamic picture: reduction in BP mainly due to reduction in TPR with maintained CO during exercise[104].

CONCLUSIONS

The haemodynamic effects and mode of action of our antihypertensive drugs differ greatly and knowledge of their mode of action is important for a rational antihypertensive therapy.

In *secondary hypertension* it is sometimes possible to cure hypertension permanently and to normalize the central haemodynamics. We observed this 10 years ago in a patient with unilateral renal artery stenosis. After removal of the stenotic kidney, the BP fell to normal values. After 1 year there was a normal TPR, CO and SV[105]. Later systematic studies in a large patient-group have shown the same results[106).

The currently available antihypertensive drugs do not always induce

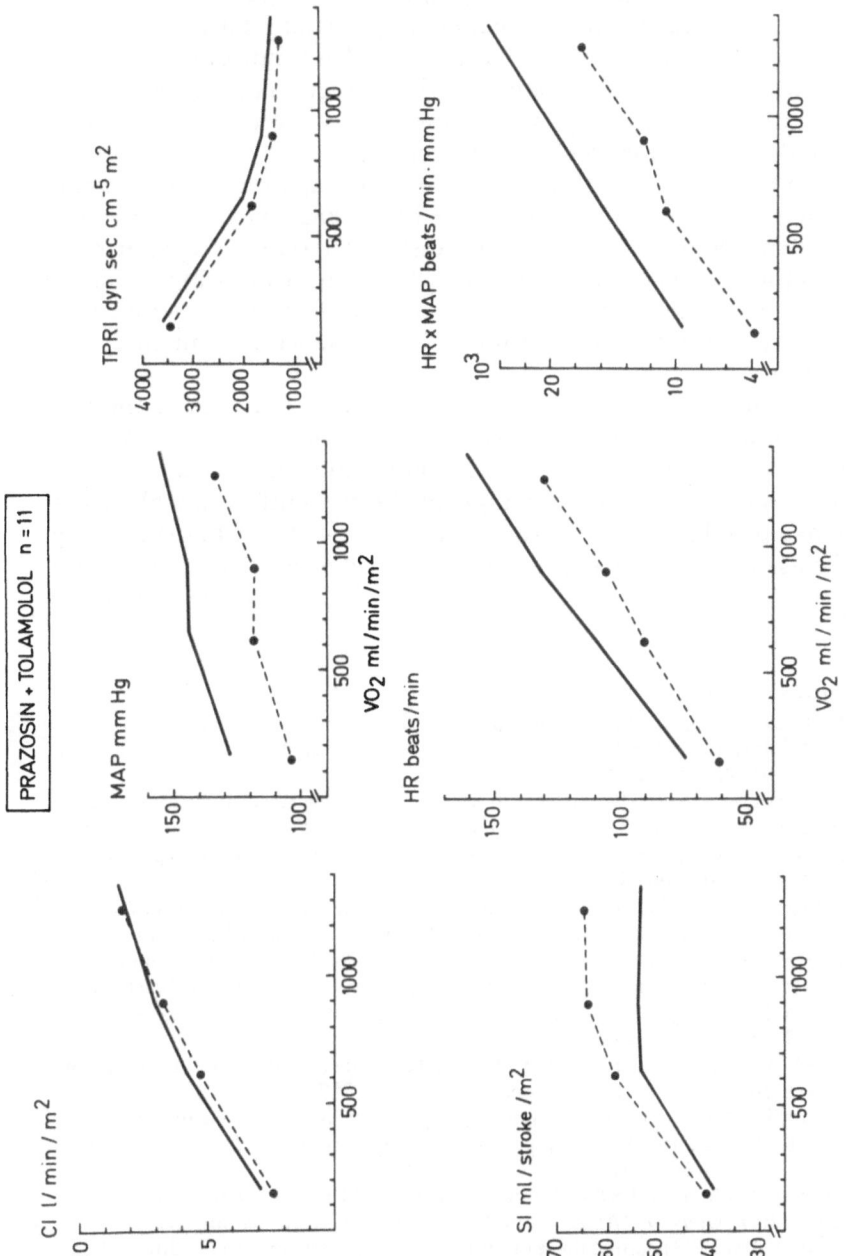

Figure 11 Haemodynamic changes induced by 1-year treatment with prazosin and tolamolol. Note the difference from the response to prazosin alone (Figure 10): the post-treatment heart rate is lower and the reduction in blood pressure greater. Legend as in Figure 1. (From Ref. 104 with kind permission from *British Journal of Clinical Pharmacology*)

the same favourable haemodynamic changes, but sometimes may replace one pathological circulatory system by another. The greatest normalization in central haemodynamics is achieved by the long-term use of thiazide diuretics and by prazosin. The beta-blockers, however, lead to a persistent decrease in CO. Nevertheless, this reduction in CO seems to be well tolerated in most patients with essential hypertension, and one might wonder if a 'normal' CO is truly necessary.

It should be emphasized that since several mechanisms seem to maintain the high BP, attempts to control the hypertension by affecting only one of these mechanisms may be unsuccessful. Therefore, polypharmacy represents the most effective approach to the treatment of hypertension today. By proper drug combinations it is often possible to induce a circulatory state which resembles the normal, and hopefully will carry the same prognosis.

A crucial question today is at what stage antihypertensive therapy should be initiated. Clinical and experimental evidence shows that it is easier to normalize the BP and the central haemodynamics in the early phase of hypertension. However, none of the presently available drugs are free of side-effects, and thus it is still undecided at what stage they should be used. Hopefully, the future will provide better and safer drugs, and make it possible to stop the vicious circle of hypertension at an early stage.

References

1 Freis, E. D. (1960). Hemodynamics of hypertension. *Physiol. Rev.*, **40**, 27
2 Lund-Johansen, P. (1967). Hemodynamics in early essential hypertension. *Acta Med. Scand.*, **482** (Suppl.), 1
3 Sannerstedt, R. (1970). Differences in haemodynamic pattern in various types of hypertension. *Triangle, The Sandoz Journal of Medical Science*, **9**, 293
4 Lund-Johansen, P. (1977). Central haemodynamics in essential hypertension. *Acta Med. Scand.*, **606** (Suppl.), 35
5 Folkow, B. (1975). Vascular changes in hypertension – review and recent animal studies. In G. Berglund, L. Hansson and L. Werkö (eds.). *Pathology and Management of Arterial Hypertension*, pp. 95–113. (Göteborg: Lindgren and Söner AB)
6 Brod, J. (1973). Regional blood flow in essential hypertension. In G. Onesti, K. E. Kim and J. H. Moyer (eds.). *Hypertension: Mechanisms and Management*, pp. 37–43. (New York: Grune and Stratton)
7 Frohlich, E. D., Tarazi, R. C. and Dustan, H. P. (1969). Re-examination of the hemodynamics of hypertension. *Amer. J. Med. Sci.*, **257**, 9
8 Frohlich, E. D. (1973). Hemodynamics of the renal hypertensions in man. In G. Onesti, K. E. Kim and J. H. Moyer (eds.). *Hypertension: Mechanisms and Management*, pp. 601-608. (New York: Grune and Stratton)
9 Birkenhäger, W. H. and Schalekamp, M. A. D. H. (1976). *Control Mechanism in Essential Hypertension*. (Amsterdam: Elsevier Scientific Publishing Company)
10 Cannon, P. J. (1973). Clinical use of diuretics in hypertension. In G. Onesti, K. E. Kim and J. H. Moyer (eds.). *Hypertension: Mechanisms and Management*, pp.

261–272. (New York: Grune and Stratton)

11 Mudge, G. H. (1976). Diuretics and other agents employed in the mobilization of edema fluid. In L. S. Goodman and A. Gilman (eds.). *The Pharmacological Basis of Therapeutics*, pp. 817–847. (New York: Macmillan Publishing Co., Inc.)

12 Peters, G. (1966). Pharmacology of diuretics. In F. Gross (ed.). *Antihypertensive Therapy – Principles and Practice*, pp. 31–57. (Berlin: Springer Verlag)

13 Beermann, B., Groschinsky-Grind, M. and Rosén, A. (1976). Absorption, metabolism and excretion of hydrochlorothiazide. *Clin. Pharmacol. Ther.*, **9**, 531

14 Crosley, A. P., Cullen, R. C., White, D., Freeman, J. F., Castillo, C. A. and Rowe, C. C. (1960). Studies of the mechanism of action of chlorothiazide in cardiac and renal disorders. *J. Lab. Clin. Med.*, **55**, 182

15 Greene, M. A., Boltax, A. J. and Scherr, E. S. (1961). Acute effects of intravenous chlorothiazide upon cardiovascular hemodynamics. *Am. Heart J.*, **62**, 659

16 Villarreal, H., Exaire, J. E., Revollo, A. and Soni, J. (1962). Effects of chlorothiazide on systemic hemodynamics in essential hypertension. *Circulation*, **26**, 405

17 Rowe, G. G., Castillo, C. A., Crosley, A. P., Maxwell, G. M. and Crumpton, C. W. (1962). Acute systemic and coronary hemodynamic effects of chlorothiazide in subjects with systemic hypertension. *Am. J. Cardiol.*, **10**, 183

18 Dustan, H., Cumming, C. R., Corcoran, A. C. and Page, I. H. (1959). A mechanism of chlorothiazide-enhanced effectiveness of antihypertensive ganglioplegic drugs. *Circulation*, **19**, 360

19 Frohlich, E. D., Schnaper, H. W., Wilson, I. M. and Freis, E. D. (1960). Hemodynamic alterations in hypertensive patients due to chlorothiazide. *N. Engl. J. Med.*, **262**, 1261

20 Conway, J. and Lauwers, P. (1960). Hemodynamic and hypotensive effects of long-term therapy with chlorothiazide. *Circulation*, **21**, 21

21 Varnauskas, E., Cramer, G., Malmcrona, R. and Werkö, L. (1961). Effect of chlorothiazide on blood pressure and blood flow at rest and on exercise in patients with arterial hypertension. *Clin. Sci.*, **20**, 406

22 Finnerty, F. A. Jr., Davidov, M. and Kakaviatos, N. (1968). Relation of sodium balance to arterial pressure during drug-induced saluresis. *Circulation*, **37**, 175

23 Eckstein, J. W., Wendling, M. G. and Abboud, F. M. (1964). Effect of prolonged treatment with chlorothiazide on cardiovascular responses to norepinephrine *J. Lab. Clin. Med.*, **64**, 853

24 Lund-Johansen, P. (1970). Hemodynamic changes in long-term diuretic therapy of essential hypertension. *Acta Med. Scand.*, **187**, 509

25 Hansen, J. (1968). Hydrochlorothiazide in the treatment of hypertension. *Acta Med. Scand.*, **183**, 317

26 Leth, A. (1970). Changes in plasma and extracellular fluid volumes in patients with essential hypertension during long-term treatment with hydrochlorothiazide. *Circulation*, **42**, 479

27 Wilson, I. M. and Freis, E. D. (1959). Relationship between plasma and extracellular fluid volume depletion and the antihypertensive effect of chlorothiazide. *Circulation*, **20**, 1028

28 Dustan, H. P., Tarazi, R. C. and Bravo, E. L. (1976). False tolerance to antihypertensive drugs. In M. P. Sambhi (ed.). *Systemic Effects of Antihypertensive Agents*, pp. 51–67. (New York: Symposia Specialists)

29 Tarazi, R. C. (1973). Diuretic drugs: Mechanisms of antihypertensive action. In G. Onesti, K. E. Kim and J. H. Moyer (eds.). *Hypertension: Mechanisms and Management*, pp. 251–260. (New York: Grune and Stratton)

30 Freis, E. D. (1976). Hemodynamic changes during acute and chronic

administration of thiazide diuretics. In M. P. Sambhi (ed.). *Systemic Effects of Antihypertensive Agents*, pp. 41–49. (New York: Symposia Specialists)

31 Sannerstedt, R. (1973). Olika medels inverkan på hemodynamiken i kort och långt perspektiv. In A. Vedin, C. Wilhelmsson and L. Werkø (eds.). *Hypertension*, pp. 248–259. (Gφteborg)

32 Danielsson, M., Bevegård, S. and Castenfors, J. (1975). Effekt på central hemodynamik under mefrusid terapi. In Bayer (Sverige) AB (ed.). *Hypertonisymposium/Saltsjφbaden*, pp. 31–36. (Uppsala: Centraltryckeriet)

33 Lewis, P. J., Kohner, E. M., Petrie, A. and Dollery, C. T. (1976). Deterioration of glucose tolerance in hypertensive patients on prolonged diuretic treatment. *Lancet*, **i**, 564

34 Atkins, L. L. (1973). Long-term use of furosemide alone in hypertension. In G. Onesti, K. E. Kim and J. H. Moyer (eds.). *Hypertension; Mechanisms and Management*, pp. 273–281. (New York: Grune and Stratton)

35 Hesse, B., Nielsen, I. and Lund-Jacobsen, H. (1975). The early effects of intravenous frusemide on central haemodynamics venous tone and plasma renin activity. *Clin. Sci. Mol. Med.*, **49**, 551

36 Ganguly, A. and Luetscher, J. A. (1976). Spironolactone therapy in primary aldosteronism: diagnostic and therapeutic implications. In M. P. Sambhi (ed.). *Systemic Effects of Antihypertensive Agents*, pp. 383–392. (New York: Symposia Specialists)

37 Weinberger, M. H. and Grim, C. E. (1976). Effects of spironolactone and hydrochlorothiazide on blood pressure and plasma renin activity in hypertension. In M. P. Sambhi (ed.). *Systemic Effects of Antihypertensive Agents*, pp. 481–493. (New York: Symposia Specialists)

38 Vaughan, E. D. Jr., Laragh, J H., Gavras, Bühler, F. R., Gavras, H., Brunner, H. R. and Baer, L. (1973). Volume factor in low and normal renin essential hypertension. *Am. J. Cardiol.*, **32**, 523

39 Bevegård, S., Castenfors, J. and Danielsson, M. (1978). The effects of four months' treatment with spironolactone on systemic blood pressure, cardiac output and plasma renin activity in hypertensive patients. *Acta Med. Scand.* (In press)

40 Laverty, R. (1973). The mechanisms of action of some antihypertensive drugs. *Br. Med. Bull.*, **29**, 152

41 Nickerson, M. and Collier, B. (1976). Drugs inhibiting adrenergic nerves and structures innervated by them. In L. S. Goodman and A. Gilman (eds.). *The Pharmacological Basis of Therapeutics*, pp. 533–564. (New York: Macmillan Publishing Co., Inc.)

42 Henning, M. (1977). New trends in pharmacology. *Acta Med. Scand.*, **606** (Suppl.), 87

43 Kwan, K. C., Foltz, E. L., Breault, G. O., Baer, J. E. and Totaro, J. A. (1976). Pharmacokinetics of methyldopa in man. *J. Pharmacol. Exp. Ther.*, **198**, 264

44 Vicet, W. A., Kašhemsant, U., Cuddy, R. P., Smulyan, H. and Eich, R. H. (1963). The acute hemodynamic effects of L-alpha methyldopa. *Am. J. Med. Sci.*, **84**, 558

45 Wilson, W. R., Fisher, F. D. and Kirkendall, W. M. (1961). The acute hemodynamic effects of alpha-methyldopa in man. *J. Chron. Dis.*, **15**, 907

46 Onesti, G., Brest, A. N., Novack, P., Kasparian, H. and Moyer, J. H. (1964). Pharmacodynamic effects of alpha-methyldopa in hypertensive subjects. *Am. Heart J.*, **67**, 32

47 Onesti, G. (1976). Systemic hemodynamic effects on alpha-methyldopa in man. In G. Onesti, M. Fernandes and K. E. Kim (eds.). *Regulation of Blood Pressure by*

the Central Nervous System, pp. 387–396. (New York: Grune and Stratton)

48 Lund-Johansen, P. (1972). Hemodynamic changes in long-term alpha-methyldopa therapy of essential hypertension. *Acta Med. Scand.*, **192,** 221

49 Dollery, C. T. and Bulpitt, C. J. (1973). Alphamethyldopa in the treatment of hypertension: Long-term experience. In G. Onesti, K. E. Kim and J. H. Moyer (eds.). *Hypertension: Mechanisms and Management*, pp. 299–304. (New York: Grune and Stratton)

50 Koghill, P. J., Smith, P. G., Benton, P., Brown, R. C. and Matthews, H. L. (1974). Methyldopa liver damage. *Br. Med. J.*, **3,** 545

51 Kobinger, W. (1973). Pharmacologic basis of the cardiovascular actions of clonidine. In G. Onesti, K. E. Kim and J. H. Moyer (eds.). *Hypertension: Mechanisms and Management*, pp. 369–380. (New York: Grune and Stratton)

52 Lund-Johansen, P. (1976). Hemodynamic effects of clonidine in man. In G. Onesti, M. Fernandes and K. E. Kim (eds.). *Regulation of Blood Pressure by the Central Nervous System*, pp. 355–365. (New York: Grune and Stratton)

53 Dollery, C. T., Davies, D. S., Draffan, G. H., Dargie, H. J., Dean, C. R., Reid, J. L., Clare, R. A. and Murray, S. (1976). Clinical pharmacology and pharmacokinetics of clonidine. *Clin. Pharmacol. Ther.*, **19,** 11

54 Safar, M., Corvol, P., Weiss, Y., Folliot, A. and Ménard, J. (1974). Action antihypertensive de trois drogues inhibant le systéme nerveux sympathique. *Nouv. Presse Med.*, **3,** 871

55 Hunyor, S. N., Hansson, L., Harrison, T. S. and Hoobler, S. W. (1973). Effects of clonidine withdrawal: Possible mechanisms and suggestions for management. *Br. Med. J.*, **11,** 209

56 Shen, D., Gibaldi, M., Throne, M., Bellward, G., Cunningham, R., Isralli, Z., Dayton, P. and McNay, J. (1975). Pharmacokinetics of bethanidine in hypertensive patients. *Clin. Pharmacol. Ther.*, **17,** 363

57 Dollery, C. T., Emslie-Smith, D. and Milne, M. D. (1960). Clinical and pharmacological studies with guanethidine in the treatment of hypertension. *Lancet*, **ii,** 381

58 Chrysant, S. G., Nishiyama, K., Adamopoulos, P. N. and Frohlich, E. D. (1975). Systemic hemodynamic effects of bethanidine in essential hypertension. *Circulation*, **52,** 137

59 Brest, A. N., Novack, P., Kasparian, H. and Moyer, J. H. (1962). Guanethidine. *Diseases of the Chest, Official Journal of the American College of Chest Physicians*, **42,** 359

60 Gifford, R. W. (1973). Reserpine and guanethidine in the treatment of hypertension. In G. Onesti, K. E. Kim and J. H. Moyer (eds.). *Hypertension: Mechanism and Management* pp. 305–309. (New York: Grune and Stratton)

61 Sannerstedt, R. and Conway, J. (1970). Hemodynamic and vascular responses to antihypertensive treatment with adrenergic blocking agents: A review. *Am. Heart J.*, **79,** 122

62 Prichard, B. N. C. and Gillam, P. M. S. (1964). The use of propranolol in the treatment of hypertension. *Br. Med. J.*, **ii,** 725

63 Birkenhäger, W. H., de Leeuw, P. W., Wester, A., Kho, T. L., Vandongen, R. and Falke, H. E. (1977). Therapeutic effects of beta-adrenoceptor blocking agents in hypertension. In P. Frick, G.-A. von Harnack, G. A. Martini, A. Prader, R. Schoen and H. P. Wolff (eds.). *Ergbnisse Inneren Medizin und Kinderheilkunde*, pp. 117–134. (Berlin: Springer Verlag)

64 Tarazi, R. C. (1973). Long-term hemodynamic effects of beta-adrenergic blockade in hypertension. In G. Onesti, K. E. Kim and J. H. Moyer (eds.).

Hypertension: Mechanisms and Management, pp. 343–349. (New York: Grune and Stratton)

65 Johnsson, G. and Regårdh, C.-G. (1976). Clinical pharmacokinetics of beta-adrenoreceptor blocking drugs. *Clin. Pharmacokin.*, **1**, 233

66 Johnsson, G., De Guzman, M., Bergman, H. and Sannerstedt, R. (1969). The haemodynamic effects of alprenolol and propranolol at rest and during exercise in hypertensive patients. *Pharmacol. Clin.*, **2**, 34

67 Hansson, L. (1973). Beta-adrenergic blockade in essential hypertension. *Acta Med. Scand.*, **550** (Suppl.), 7

68 Sannerstedt, R. (1975). Haemodynamic effects of adrenergic beta-receptor-blocking agents in arterial hypertension. In G. Berglund, L. Hansson and L. Werkö (eds.). *Pathophysiology and Management of Arterial Hypertension*, pp. 194–200. (Gotebörg: Lindgren and Söner AB)

69 Tarzi, R. C. and Dustan, H. P. (1972). Beta-adrenergic blockade in hypertension. *Am. J. Cardiol.*, **29**, 633

70 Ulrych, M., Frohlich, E. D., Dustan, H. P. and Page, I. H. (1968). Immediate hemodynamic effects of beta-adrenergic blockade with propranolol in normotensive and hypertensive man. *Circulation*, **37**, 411

71 Franciosa, J. A., Freis, E. D. and Conway, J, (1973). Antihypertensive and hemodynamic properties of the new beta adrenergic blocking agent timolol. *Circulation*, **48**, 118

72 Frohlich, E. D., Tarazi, R. C., Dustan, H. P. and Page, I. H. (1968). The paradox of beta-adrenergic blockade in hypertension. *Circulation*, **37**, 417

73 Lydtin, H., Kusus, T., Daniel, W., Schierl, W., Ackenheil, M., Kempter, H., Lohmoller, G., Niklas, M. and Walter, I.(1972). Propranolol therapy in essential hypertension. *Am. Heart J.*, **83**, 589

74 Glezer, G. A., Moskalenko, N. P., Megrelishvili, R. I. and Zilbert, N. L. (1976). Effects of propranolol on haemodynamic changes and gas exchange at rest, in orthostasis, and on exercise in patients with arterial hypertension. *Cor Vasa*, **18**, 26

75 Lund-Johansen, P. (1976). Hemodynamic long-term effects of timolol at rest and during exercise in essential hypertension. *Acta Med. Scand.*, **109**, 263

76 Aronow, W. S., Ferlinz, J., Del Vicario, M., Moorthy, K., King, J. and Cassidy, J. (1976). Effect of timolol versus propranolol on hypertension and hemodynamics. *Circulation*, **54**, 47

77 Lund-Johansen, P. (1974). Hemodynamic changes at rest and during exercise in long-term beta-blocker therapy of essential hypertension. *Acta Med. Scand.*, **195**, 117

78 Atterhög, J.-H., Dunér, H. and Pernow, B. (1977). Haemodynamic effects of pindolol in hypertensive patients. *Acta Med. Scand.*, **606** (Suppl.), 55

79 Reybrouck, T., Amery, A. and Billiet, L. (1977). Hemodynamic response to graded exercise after chronic beta-adrenergic blockade. *J. Appl. Physiol.*, **42**, 133

80 Lund-Johansen, P. (1976). Hemodynamic long-term effects of a new beta-blocker atenolol (ICI 66082). *Br. J. Clin. Pharmacol.*, **3**, 445

81 Lund-Johansen, P. and Ohm, O.-J. (1977). Hemodynamic long-term effects of metoprolol at rest and during exercise in essential hypertension. *Br. J. Clin. Pharmacol.*, **4**, 147

82 Trap-Jensen, J., Clausen, J. P., Noer, I., Larsen, O. A., Krogsgaard, A. R. and Christensen, N. J. (1976). The effects of beta-adrenoceptor blockers on cardiac output, liver blood flow and skeletal muscle blood flow in hypertensive patients. *Acta Physiol. Scand.*, **440** (Suppl.), 30

83 Lambert, D. M. D. (1974). Hypertension and myocardial infarction. *Br. Med. J.*, **3**, 685
84 Vedin, J. A. and Wilhelmsson, C. E. (1975). Long-term postinfarction treatment with practolol. *Bri. Med. J.*, **4**, 579
85 Taylor, S. H., Sutherland, G. R., MacKenzie, G. J., Staunton, H. P. and Donald, K. W. (1965). The circulatory effects of intravenous phentolamine in man. *Circulation*, **31**, 741
86 Vlackhakis, N. D. and Mendlowitz, M. (1976). Alpha- and beta-adrenergic receptor blocking agents combined with a diuretic in the treatment of essential hypertension. *J. Clin. Pharmacol.*, **16**, 352
87 Beilin, L. H. and Juel-Jensen, B. E. (1972). Alpha and beta adrenergic blockade in hypertension. *Lancet*, **i**, 979
88 Martin, L. E., Hopkins, R. and Bland, R. (1976). Metabolism of labetalol by animals and man. *Br. J. Clin. Pharmacol.*, **3** (Suppl.), 695
89 Koch, G. (1976). Haemodynamic effects of combined alpha- and beta-adrenoceptor blockade after intravenous labetalol in hypertensive patients at rest and during exercise. *Br. J. Clin. Pharmacol.*, **3** (Suppl.), 725
90 Lund-Johansen, P. and Bakke, O. M. (1978). Haemodynamic effects and plasma concentrations of labetalol during long-term treatment of essential hypertension. *Br. J. Clin. Pharmacol.* (In press)
91 Rønne-Rasmussen, J. O., Andersen, G. S., Bowal Jensen, N. and Andersson, E. (1976). Acute effect of intravenous labetalol in the treatment of systemic arterial hypertension. *Br. J. Clin. Pharmacol.*, **3** (Suppl.), 805
92 Ablad, B. (1963). A study of the mechanism of the hemodynamic effects of hydralazine in man. *Acta Pharmacol. Toxicol.*, **1** (Suppl.), 1
93 Nickerson, M. and Ruedy, J. (1976). Antihypertensive agents and the drug therapy of hypertension. In L. S. Goodman and A. Gilman (eds.). *The Pharmacological basis of Therapeutics*, pp. 705–726. (New York: Macmillan Publishing Co., Inc.)
94 Koch-Weser, J. (1976). Drug therapy. Hydralazine. *N. Engl. J. Med.*, **295**, 320
95 Constantine, J. W. (1974). Analysis of the hypotensive action of prazosin. In D. W. K. Cotton (ed.). *Prazosin – Evaluation of a New Antihypertensive Agent*, pp. 16–36. (Amsterdam: Excerpta Medica)
96 Smith, I. S., Fernandes, M., Kim, K. E., Swartz, C. and Onesti, G. (1975). A three-phase clinical evaluation of prazosin. *Prazosin – Clinical Symposium Proceedings*, pp. 53–60. (New York: McGraw Hill)
97 Lund-Johansen, P. (1974). Haemodynamic changes at rest and during exercise in long-term prazosin therapy of essential hypertension. In D. W. K. Cotton (ed.). *Prazosin – Evaluation of a new Antihypertensive Agent*, pp. 43–53. (Amsterdam: Excerpta Medica)
98 Mroczek, W. J., Leibel, B. A., Davidov, M. and Finnerty, F. A. Jr. (1971). The importance of the rapid administration of diazoxide in accelerated hypertension. *N. Engl. J. Med.*, **285**, 603
99 Bhatia, S. K. and Frohlich, E. D. (1973). Hemodynamic comparison of agents useful in hypertensive emergencies. *Am. Heart J.*, **85**, 367
100 Bryan, R. K., Hoobler, S. W., Rosenzweig, J. and Weller, J. M. (1977). Effect of minoxidil on blood pressure and hemodynamics in severe hypertension. *Am. J. Cardiol.*, **39**, 796
101 Kaplan, N. M., Bryan Holland, O. and Gomez-Sanchez, C. (1976). Effects of antihypertensive therapy on plasma renin activity. In M. P. Sambhi (ed.). *Systemic Effects of Antihypertensive Agents*, pp. 207–216. (New York: Symposia

Specialists)
102 Sannerstedt, R., Stenberg, J., Johnsson, G. and Werkø, L. (1971). Hemodynamic interference of alprenolol with dihydralazine in normal and hypertensive man. *Am. J. Cardiol.*, **28**, 316
103 Hansson, L., Olander, R., Aberg, H., Malmcrona, R. and Westerlund, A. (1971). Treatment of hypertension with propranolol and hydralazine. *Acta Med. Scand.*, **190**, 531
104 Lund-Johansen, P. (1977). Haemodynamic long-term effects of prazosin plus tolamolol in essential hypertension. *Br. J. Clin. Pharmacol.*, **4**, 141
105 Lund-Johansen, P. (1968). Diureticaterapi ved moderat essensiell hypertensjon fra hemodynamisk synspunkt. *Farmakoterapi*, **24**, 65
106 Tarazi, R. C., Frohlich, E. D. and Dustan, H. P. (1973). Contribution of cardiac output to renovascular hypertension in man. *Am. J. Cardiol.*, **31**, 600

5

How to treat essential hypertension

M. Moser

THE ART OF THERAPY: AN IMPORTANT FIRST STEP

The interrelationship between the science and art of medicine is most apparent in the management of hypertension, a disease where patients do not usually seek medical care because of a symptom. In most instances, a diagnosis is imposed upon an apparently healthy individual. He is then given medication and simultaneously informed that certain lifestyle changes may be necessary, or that some of the medication might make him feel unwell. The scientist–physician who undertakes therapy, based upon facts and a good prospect of decreasing morbidity and prolonging life, must, above all, be a sympathetic but firm therapist and a skilful health educator with patience over a long period of time in order to overcome some of these problems. Before undertaking the treatment of any hypertensive patient, therefore, a solid relationship between the therapist, whether a physician, nurse practitioner, or other health-care provider, must be established. This process will often take some time but, when measured within the total context of years of therapy, will be time well spent. Elsewhere (Chapter 7) Dr Finnerty has summarized some techniques that he has found useful in gaining and maintaining patient adherence to therapy. Unless the therapist is able to accomplish this, long-term management will not succeed, regardless of the method of treatment chosen.

WHICH PATIENTS SHOULD BE TREATED?

In Chapter 1 Dr Freis has discussed the risks of elevated blood pressure, noting that the higher the pressure, the greater the risk of cardiovascular complications; the more evidence of target-organ involvement, the higher the risk; the greater the degree of renal insufficiency, the greater the risk. These are some factors that help in reaching a conclusion about

93

whom to treat and with what degree of urgency. The presence of other risk factors for cardiovascular disease, such as a high blood cholesterol level or the presence of diabetes, *and* a knowledge of the results that might be expected from long-term blood-pressure lowering with antihypertensive drug therapy in specific cases must also be considered in planning a treatment programme[1,2].

A decision regarding the levels of blood pressure that constitute hypertension is of primary importance – such definitions are obviously arbitrary. Based upon epidemiological data, a blood pressure of 140/90 mmHg or higher on at least two occasions in a patient aged 50 years or younger may be considered significantly elevated to require follow-up and probably therapy[3]. In patients aged 50 years or older, some investigators do not believe that a diagnosis of hypertension and specific treatment are justified unless the blood pressure is 160/95 mmHg or higher. There is no question that these levels carry an increased risk, but the elevated pressure, especially the systolic readings in older patients, may reflect 'arteriosclerotic' changes in large blood vessels, and prognosis may not be influenced by blood pressure lowering; hence, they argue, 'why treat the patient and expose him to possible side-effects?'

AN APPROACH TO THERAPY

In the recently released USA Joint National Committee Report on Detection, Evaluation and Treatment of High Blood Pressure[4], reasonable guidelines for initiating therapy are outlined (Table 1 – modified from the Joint National Report). The decision regarding the urgency of treatment will obviously depend upon the height of the blood pressure and the presence or absence of target-organ changes; i.e., if the blood pressure is 210/120 mmHg and left ventricular hypertrophy is present, the decision to use antihypertensive drugs, and use them in full dosages, is an easy one to arrive at. However, in the patient with borderline elevations of blood pressure, such as 140/90 to 150/95 mmHg, in the 40–45 year age group, an attempt to utilize other methods of therapy may be warranted.

In Chapter 3 Dr Gifford has summarized the work-up of the hypertensive patient prior to instituting therapy. In view of recently reported data suggesting that secondary forms of the disease are even less common than previously believed (probably under 1%)[5], we agree with his and the Joint National Committee Report's conclusions that a simple diagnostic evaluation, without resort to extensive testing or expensive hospitalization, is appropriate in the vast majority of cases. Therapy, and not the diagnostic work-up, should be stressed. Too often physicians

Table 1 **Guidelines for initiating therapy in patients with elevated blood pressure***

Average diastolic blood pressure	*Recommended action*
120 or higher	Immediate evaluation and treatment indicated
105–119	Treatment indicated
90–104	Individualize treatment (see Table 3)
Under 90	Re-measure blood pressure at yearly intervals

Repeat or confirmation blood pressures are recommended whenever the previous initial measurement reveals either a blood pressure level of 140/99 mmHg or higher in a person under age 50 or 160/95 mmHg in all persons.

* Adapted from Joint National Committee Report on Detection, Evaluation and Treatment of High Blood Pressure[4].

believe that their obligation to the patient has been fulfilled by an exhaustive evaluation.

One of many cases observed by us through the years that illustrates this problem of a 'so-called excellent' diagnostic approach with poor therapy is that of a 56-year-old lawyer whose blood pressure was found to be elevated to levels of 150–160/100 mmHg at age 48. He was followed for several years without therapy, but when pressures rose to 200–220/120–130 mmHg, he was referred for study. A complete in-patient evaluation, over a 5-day period, was done, including an intravenous urogram, repeated urinary and serum electrolytes, renin determinations, careful studies of renal function and catecholamine excretion. He was discharged from the hospital and reassured that no cause had been found for his high blood pressure. His physician was warned not to use excessive amounts of diuretics or other potent blood pressure lowering drugs because of a decreased creatinine clearance and a serum creatinine level of 2·5 mg%. Little or no therapy was given; blood pressures remained at 220–240/130–140 mmHg.

When first seen by us 1 year later, and 4 years after the initial discovery of a mild elevation of blood pressure, he had grade II fundi, left ventricular hypertrophy, and a creatinine of 3·5 mg% – well on his way to renal failure and eventual dialysis. On appropriate therapy, which included one tablet a day of a chlorthalidone–reserpine combination, plus 200 mg/day (4 tablets) of hydralazine and 37½ mg/day (1½ tablets) of guanethidine, blood pressure control was achieved. He has been followed for the past 3 years; blood pressures are normal, left ventricular hypertrophy is no longer present, and serum creatinine levels are between 1·8 and 2·4 mg%. His prognosis is good, but how much better it might have been had therapy been started before evidence of target-organ damage was noted.

After a simple but careful evaluation has been carried out, a decision regarding the specific type of treatment to lower blood pressure must be made.

The role of diet in treatment

(a)   Although it is well known that a diet containing less than 500 mg of sodium a day will lower blood pressure[6], even in patients with severe accelerated or malignant hypertension, this type of rigid dietary management is rarely used in therapy. It is impractical for the majority of hypertensive patients; nor would many patients remain on such a diet for long periods of time even though they might be aware of the significant risk of elevated blood pressure. In the very few highly motivated patients who can tolerate this form of treatment, blood pressure lowering will occur in a fairly high percentage of cases.

Will moderate restriction of salt lower blood pressure? There are some data from studies of Parijs[7] that a moderate reduction of salt intake from the usual 10–12 g/day, which is the average American intake, to a level of 4–5 g/day will lower blood pressure in the patient with mild or moderately severe hypertension, when diet therapy is the sole method of treatment. This degree of restriction can be accomplished by: (1) reducing the intake of processed foods, such as frankfurters and frozen vegetables; (2) eliminating pretzels, peanuts, and other obviously heavily salted foods, such as bacon and pickles, from the diet; (3) reducing the use of table salt; and (4) using herbs, pepper and other non-sodium-containing condiments in cooking. A great many people can tolerate this degree of salt restriction if reasons for the programme are carefully explained. Possibly some patients with mild hypertension can be managed successfully by this approach although controlled data are obviously needed. A sample diet list that we have used as part of a patient instruction booklet is reproduced in Table 2.

On the other hand, there is some evidence that a high salt intake of more than 15–20 g daily will decrease the effectiveness of diuretic therapy when these medications are utilized to lower blood pressure[8]. It is probably prudent, therefore, to urge every hypertensive patient to remain on as low a sodium intake as he can tolerate without making his life miserable or turning the household into a 'diet kitchen'. It is, however, a mistake to depend solely on a low-salt diet as therapy in patients with moderate or severe hypertension, i.e., levels of greater than 180/110 mmHg and evidence of target-organ involvement, such as left ventricular hypertrophy. Most of the time, this approach does not work!

Some investigators have advocated both salt and carbohydrate restriction in the management of hypertension[9]. A low carbohydrate intake will decrease the amount of salt absorbed from the small bowel, and will

Table 2   Foods with high salt content

Potato chips	Bouillon
Pretzels	Ham
Salted crackers	Sausages
Biscuits	Frankfurters
Pancakes	Smoked meats or fish
Pastries or cakes made from self-rising flour mixes	Sardines
	Tomato juice, canned
Pickles	Lima beans, frozen
Sauerkraut	Peas, frozen
Soy sauce	Spinach, canned
Catsup	Carrots, canned
Olives	Many kinds of cheese
Commercially prepared soups or stews	

This table lists foods with a high salt or sodium content that should be avoided or limited if you have high blood pressure. In general, it is a good idea to use little or no salt at the table or in food preparation. Use paprika, pepper, oregano, cloves, cinnamon, or lemon juice instead. Avoid foods that are obviously salty or preserved in salt or brine.

also increase sodium excretion by the kidneys, but patients must discipline themselves severely to follow this regimen, and most patients are unable to do this. Generally, patient adherence to therapy will be decreased if drastic lifestyle changes are attempted.

(*b*) Obesity has been linked with hypertension. Hypertensive patients, both adults and children, are frequently obese, and obese patients are frequently hypertensive[10]. Because of this association, weight reduction is often considered a prime method of treating hypertension. While it is true that significant reduction of weight in obese patients will occasionally reduce blood pressure in mild to moderately severe hypertension, it is an all-too-frequent error in therapy to depend solely upon weight reduction as definitive therapy. Frequently an obese hypertensive patient is placed on a weight reduction programme and followed carefully, only to realize that 6 months to 1 year after the diet is instituted, little or no progress has been made. The patient is frustrated, the physician is annoyed, the patient–doctor relationship has been strained considerably, and the blood pressure has not been lowered. In our experience, it is better practice to treat the blood pressure, as we would do in other patients, with specific antihypertensive drugs and, at the same time, do everything possible to promote weight reduction. If, in the course of 6 months to a year, the patient's weight is reduced significantly, antihypertensive drugs can always be reduced or eliminated in an attempt to see whether or not normotensive levels can be maintained without them. Time has not been lost, and the elevated blood pressure has been effectively treated. *Far too many patients are being treated by*

*weight reduction alone; blood pressure remains high and complications
occur.*

A prudent diet should be advised for all patients, thin or heavy, especially those with elevated serum cholesterol or triglyceride levels. Proof that alteration of this risk factor decreases the incidence of heart attacks has not as yet been forthcoming, but in view of extensive epidemiological data, an attempt to reduce saturated dietary fats makes sense. This can usually be done by reducing the patient's intake of dairy products and fatty meats, stressing an increased intake of fish, poultry and veal, margarine, skimmed milk, etc. Here too, diet restrictions need not be rigid except in very high-risk patients.

Obviously, newer techniques must be sought to more effectively alter the eating habits of Americans, especially with regard to total calorie, fat and salt intake. Some progress has been made, with a decrease in per capita consumption of animal fats and oils of over 50%, and of butter, eggs, and milk of between 12 and 30%, over the past 12 years, but more should be done.

BEHAVIOURAL MODIFICATION TECHNIQUES, TRANSCENDENTAL MEDITATION, BIOFEEDBACK: DO THEY HAVE A PLACE IN THERAPY?

There is evidence that transcendental meditation will lower blood pressure, decrease heart and respiratory rate, and decrease oxygen consumption during the period that the patient is meditating[11]. There are testimonial data to show that lowering of blood pressure will persist in some patients who meditate regularly. This technique is experimental, however; the data are conflicting; and whatever effects on blood pressure are noted are not of sufficient magnitude to risk the use of this technique as definitive therapy in patients with significant elevations of blood pressure[12]. The danger of total dependence upon this technique is that the patient and the physician are deluded into believing that specific therapy is being given.

The above comments also apply to various types of behavioural modification techniques and psychotherapy. Here, too, blood pressure will be lowered transiently in many instances, but the process is often a long, tedious and expensive one, and long-term blood pressure lowering by these experimental techniques has not been demonstrated. At present, patients and physicians should not depend upon them as definitive therapy.

OTHER CONSIDERATIONS IN A THERAPEUTIC PROGRAMME

(*a*)   Should the hypertensive patient be advised not to drink alcoholic beverages? There is some evidence, although not definitive, that blood pressure is highter in patients with an alcohol intake in excess of 3–4 drinks of 80 proof whiskey, 8–12 ounces of table wine, or 4–6 bottles of beer per day, than in more moderate or non-drinkers. There is no evidence, however, that the moderate intake of alcohol will influence the course of the patient with hypertension, either adversely or positively. An occasional cocktail is certainly permissible. Patients who are being treated with drugs, such as guanethidine, that reduce cardiac output as a result of venous pooling should be warned not to take more than one or two drinks at any one time, especially if they remain standing or are in a hot room, etc. Additional vasodilatation in these patients may cause syncope. (*b*) *Cigarette smoking* is recognized as one of the three major risk factors of cardiovascular disease, and all hypertensive patients should be told not to smoke, for this reason[13]. 'Chain smoking' will elevate blood pressure as a result of catecholamine release and a direct vasoconstrictor effect of nicotine on blood vessels. Increase in heart rate and cardiac work also occurs in chain smokers. However, an occasional cigarette, pipe or cigar will usually have very little effect upon heart-rate, cardiac work, or blood pressure. If a patient cannot stop smoking altogether, it may be prudent to compromise and suggest pipe or cigar smoking, which carries less risk. Here again, insisting on too many lifestyle changes may lose the patient or lead him to stop all therapy.

THE USE OF TRANQUILLIZERS AND SEDATIVES

Unfortunately many physicians still depend upon the use of tranquillizers or sedatives to lower blood pressure, frequently along with weight reduction. In patients with 'labile' hypertension or elevations of blood pressure, as a result of 'anxiety episodes', blood pressure will often be lowered during these episodes by the use of these medications. However, there is little place for tranquillizers as definitive therapy in a patient with significantly elevated blood pressure. Control trials actually indicate that phenobarbital is no more effective than a placebo in the long-term management of hypertension[14,15]. If a patient is over-anxious or tense, or has insomnia that interferes with normal activities, the use of tranquillizers or sedatives for limited periods of time may be helpful; they should not be depended upon as specific antihypertensive therapy.

BASIC PRINCIPLES OF ANTIHYPERTENSIVE DRUG THERAPY; TREATMENT TO A GOAL

In recent surveys of clinics where hypertensive patients are being treated, it has been noted that only approximately 50–60% of all patients who attend the clinics, who are taking specific antihypertensive therapy, and who are reliable and 'adherent' to treatment programmes, are controlled at normotensive levels. A recent private practice audit demonstrated that the percentages are similar, except in a practice specializing in cardiology and hypertension where over 80% of patients were controlled[16]. Frequently good control is not achieved because the physician is reluctant to titrate therapy to a defined end-point. Treatment should be defined as the lowering of blood pressure to normotensive or near normotensive levels if at all possible. When queried, most physicians will answer, 'I treat all of my hypertensive patients'. When records are analysed, however, it is found that *some* therapy is being given but specific end-points are not being achieved in large numbers of patients. Some patients, i.e. elderly patients with cerebrovascular disease, may not be able to tolerate normotensive levels, but most individuals will adjust well. 'Treatment' may include as little as one dose of 50 mg of hydrochlorothiazide or chlorthalidone three or four times a week, or as many as 20–25 pills or four or five different drugs a day.

After the patient has been given the basic facts about hypertension, about the necessity for continuation of therapy, and about the possibility of side-effects, antihypertensive drug therapy should be undertaken. We have utilized several booklets effectively for patient education over the past 25 years for example, *How You Can Help Your Doctor Treat Your High Blood Pressure,* available from local American Heart Associations; and *High Blood Pressure And What You Can Do About It,* available from the Benjamin Company, 485 Madison Ave., New York, NY.

ANTIHYPERTENSIVE DRUG THERAPY

In Chapter 4 the haemodynamic effects of antihypertensive drugs have been summarized by Dr Lund-Johansen. It is apparent that medications are available that have an impact on most of the physiological variables presently believed to be important in the genesis of human hypertension: extracellular fluid volume, cardiac output, and peripheral resistance. A wide choice is available to the practising physician, with newer agents on the horizon.

The USA Joint National Committee Report recommends the use of diuretics as the Step 1 drugs of choice in the vast majority of hypertensive patients[4]. I agree with this recommendation. These drugs act to reduce extracellular fluid volume (ECF); on prolonged use, peripheral resistance is decreased. Since the use of almost all of the other antihypertensive drugs will result in some expansion of ECF with resultant 'pseudotolerance' in many patients, the use of diuretics also serves to prevent this occurrence.

Some physicians believe that a beta-adrenergic blocker should be the first drug of choice, especially in patients with a rapid heart rate, with angina, or in those with so-called 'hyperdynamic' circulations. In some of these patients, a satisfactory blood pressure response *is* obtained with propranolol alone; but even in the less severe hypertensives, only about 50% of patients respond[17]. Propranolol dosage must be titrated, the process requires several to many office or clinic visits, and as many as four to eight pills must be taken per day (160–480 mg/day); this, plus the possible cost of 40–80 cents/day versus 10–15 cents/day when a diuretic is used, are reasons against advocating this drug as Step 1 therapy except in specific instances. In the few individuals who cannot tolerate diuretics (i.e., patients with severe photosensitivity, etc.), propranolol is an acceptable Step 1 drug. Even in patients with angina and hypertension, where beta-blockade is especially useful, propranolol should probably not be used without a diuretic. When diuretic drugs are given alone, only one, or at most two, pills a day are necessary, titration can be accomplished quickly in one or two visits, and the blood pressure response rate is approximately the same or slightly higher than with a beta-blocker alone.

Method of drug titration (Tables 3 and 4)

If blood pressure levels are only moderately elevated, 140/90–160/105 mmHg for example, and the patient is asymptomatic, with no evidence of target-organ involvement, the use of a diuretic, such as hydrochlorothiazide (50 mg) or methyclothiazide (5 mg), four or five times a week, or chlorthalidone (50 mg) three times a week, may be all that is necessary to restore blood pressure to normal levels. In these instances, the patient can be seen within 1–2 months after therapy is begun and dosage adjusted according to blood pressure response. If blood pressure has not been reduced, dosage is increased, as noted, to either 50–100 mg/day of hydrochlorothiazide, 5–10 mg/day of methyclothiazide, or 50 mg/day of chlorthalidone. If blood pressure is controlled at normotensive levels 1–2 months later, the patient should be advised to have his pressure checked three to four times a year (as recommended in the Joint National Committee Report on Detection, Evaluation and Treatment of High Blood Pressure).

If blood pressure is not at normal levels on a full dose of a diuretic, the addition of a rauwolfia drug as a Step 2 drug may be indicated. Diuretics and rauwolfia may be given in a combination tablet; for example, Diupres (hydrochlorothiazide and reserpine) or Rauzide (bendroflumethiazide and rauwolfia) or Regroton (reserpine and chlorthalidone), allowing for a lesser number of pills/day and less cost. The patient often

Table 3   Recommended antihypertensive regimens*

Group 1 (90–104 mmHg)	Group 2 (105–129 mmHg)	Group 3 (≥ 130 mmHg)
Individualized therapy: possible drug therapy and/or life style changes	Step 1 Thiazide diuretics	Urgent May require hospitalization

Factors to consider:
  Male sex
  Smoking habits
  Elevated blood cholesterol
	Step 2†
	add propranolol or
	  methyldopa or
	  reserpine
		May require several drugs simultaneously
		Blood pressure levels should not be used as the sole indicator for parenteral or emergency therapy

Family history of complications Diabetes	Step 3‡ add hydralazine	
Presence of target organ damage Elevated systolic pressure	Step 4 add or substitute guanethidine	

* Adapted from the Joint National Committee Report on Detection, Evaluation and Treatment of High Blood Pressure.

* Tranquillizers and sedatives are not effective in lowering blood pressure and should not be used as primary therapy.

† Clonidine is a moderately potent antihypertensive agent which may be substituted for a Step 2 drug.

‡ Prazosin may be substituted for hydralazine.

Virtually all patients with a diastolic pressure of 105 mmHg or higher should be treated with antihypertensive drugs.

feels that his illness is less severe if he is given fewer pills to take. Combination therapy with a rauwolfia–thiazide medication is effective in over 80% of patients with mild to moderate hypertension[17].

Another Step 2 drug is propranolol, or another beta-adrenergic blocker. This medication can be added to the thiazide diuretics if the diuretics alone are ineffective. Propranolol is started at 40 mg twice daily and adjusted 1 month later to 80 mg twice daily or 40 mg four times daily if needed; it is then gradually increased at 1–2 month intervals to a total dose of 480 mg/day if necessary to reduce blood pressure to normal. This combination will also be effective in over 80% of patients with mild to moderate hypertension[17]. Although much larger doses have been given, their effectiveness has not been confirmed, and such regimens are cumbersome and expensive.

In patients where a rauwolfia–thiazide or propranolol–thiazide regimen is ineffective, the addition of hydralazine, in dosages of 25 mg twice daily initially, with increases of up to 200 mg or 250 mg/day in two div-

Table 4 Therapeutic regimen

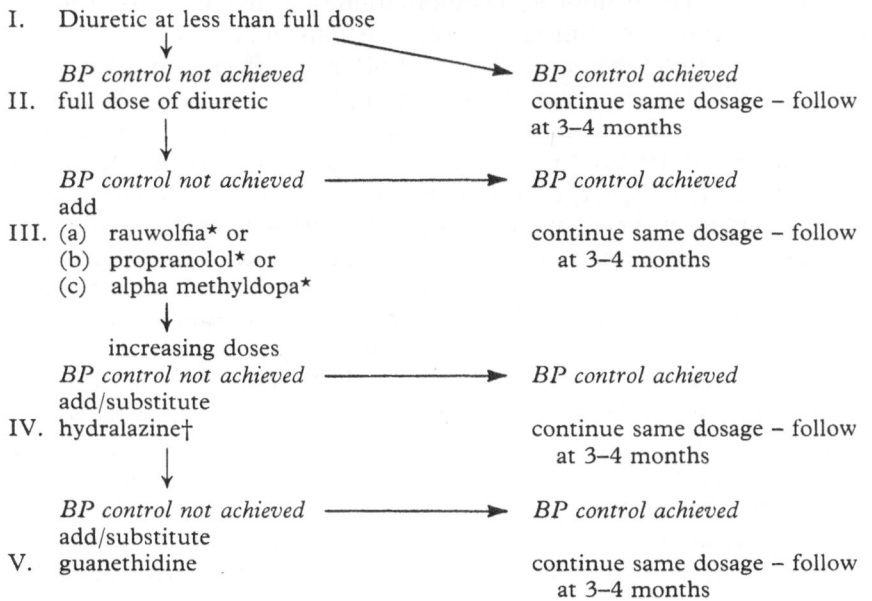

I.   Diuretic at less than full dose

    BP control not achieved   *BP control achieved*

II. full dose of diuretic   continue same dosage – follow
                                              at 3–4 months

    BP control not achieved   *BP control achieved*
    add

III. (a) rauwolfia* or   continue same dosage – follow
    (b) propranolol* or   at 3–4 months
    (c) alpha methyldopa*

    increasing doses
    BP control not achieved   *BP control achieved*
    add/substitute

IV. hydralazine†   continue same dosage – follow
                                              at 3–4 months

    BP control not achieved   *BP control achieved*
    add/substitute

V.   guanethidine   continue same dosage – follow
                                              at 3–4 months

* Clonidine may be substituted for any one of these medications.
† Prazosin may be substituted.

ided doses, will increase the percentage of patients who respond. Approximately 90% of all patients with mild to moderate hypertension will probably be controlled on this regimen.

The use of alpha-methyldopa in dosages of 250 mg twice daily, with a gradual increase to as much as 2 g/day, is another option for the physician if the patient has not responded to diuretic therapy alone. If alpha-methyldopa in the above doses is ineffective, it should be stopped and another Step 2 drug substituted or hydralazine added to the treatment programme. A combination of alpha-methyldopa and a thiazide (Aldoril) is also available. This can be used if the doses are appropriate once titration has been accomplished. Fewer pills are therefore necessary, and cost of care may be reduced. Obviously, the problem of treatment would be much simpler if we had one pill that combined three or four different ingredients, was effective in most cases, caused few side-effects, and was long-acting. Unfortunately, such a medication is not available.

In patients who present with higher diastolic blood pressures, greater than 105 mmHg, with evidence of target-organ involvement, such as left ventricular hypertrophy, there is obviously a greater urgency to lower the blood pressure. In these patients, diuretics are started with a full dosage or, in some instances, a combination of a thiazide with a Step 2 drug might represent 'initial' therapy. A rauwolfia–thiazide combination (one or two tablets per day) will often be effective even in these patients. *Initial* therapy with propranolol plus a thiazide is also appropriate, as is thiazide with alpha-methyldopa. Fewer visits are necessary if two drugs are started simultaneously; thiazides alone are usually not effective with these higher levels of blood pressure. The second drug (rauwolfia, propranolol) or alpha-methyldopa can always be withdrawn later if blood pressure is controlled, to determine whether a good result can be maintained with a diuretic alone. Patients should be seen within 1–2 weeks; more frequently than those with a lesser degree of blood pressure elevation. If, after several visits, a fall in blood pressure has not occurred, or blood pressure has not been lowered to a goal level, the addition of hydralazine in gradually increasing doses is indicated. If normotensive levels are not achieved on this regimen within 2–3 months, propranolol may be substituted for rauwolfia, or rauwolfia for propranolol, depending upon which combination was used initially. Alpha-methyldopa may also be substituted if the above combinations are ineffective. In our experience, 60–70% of these moderately severe hypertensive patients will respond to this regimen.

In patients who do not achieve normotensive or near-normotensive levels of blood pressure on the above regimen, guanethidine in gradually increasing doses may be added or substituted for alpha-methyldopa or propranolol. One-half of a 25 mg tablet can be given once daily with dosage increments every 1–2 weeks, depending upon the severity of the blood pressure, until the patient either complains of early morning dizziness or light-headedness on exercise, or until the standing blood pressure is reduced to normal levels.

There will be some patients who will respond to thiazides, propranolol and hydralazine, and others who will respond to alpha-methyldopa plus a thiazide plus hydralazine, or to thiazides rauwolfia hydralazine and guanethidine. *No one drug or combination will work in all patients*; the physician should not become rigid in his approach to therapy but must add and/or substitute different medications until blood pressure is lowered to normal levels. Once control is achieved, it is appropriate for patients to be seen every 3–4 months.

Clonidine and prazosin are other moderately potent antihypertensive drugs. Clonidine may be used or substituted for any of the Step 2 drugs; a vasodilator, prazosin, whose effect is probably the result of a central action may be used instead of hydralazine. Clonidine titration is accomplished by starting with 0·1 mg daily and increasing by 0·1 or 0·2 mg at each visit. We have not used dosages higher than 0·8 mg/day. Prazosin is started with a small dose of 1·0 mg, preferably given at night, and increased at each visit by increments of 1·0–2·0 mg to a total of 10·0–15·0 mg daily.

The question of what constitutes an adequate dosage of a specific medication is often raised. Table 5 lists suggested and maximum dosages of commonly used antihypertensive drugs. Certain drugs, such as the diuretics, have a dose–response curve which flattens out at a certain level; i.e., if 150 mg of hydrochlorothiazide is not effective, higher doses will either not significantly increase sodium excretion or lower blood pressure. Other drugs, such as guanethidine, may lower blood pressures in doses of 10 mg/day or may not be effective until dosages of 200–250 mg/day are reached. The limiting factors in this case are: (1) reaching a goal of normotensive blood pressures in the upright position, or (2) side-effects. Propranolol presents another problem concerning dosage levels. Some investigators believe that many so-called resistant patients will respond if doses are increased to 2–3 g/day. Most American physicians will not use dosages above 480 mg/day; not necessarily because larger doses produce significantly more side-effects but because of: (1) cost of therapy, and (2) the total number of pills required and the question of 'compliance'.

In general, dosages of medications should be increased within the guidelines in Table 5 until blood pressure is lowered to the desired level – a goal of normotensive or near normotensive levels, or side-effects prevent further titration.

THE PROBLEM OF SIDE-EFFECTS

Side-effects of antihypertensive drugs may represent hypersensitivity reactions, such as the 'lupus syndrome', to high doses of hydralazine, or the relatively rare photosensitivity reaction to the thiazides, or exaggerated physiological responses, such as diarrhoea or postural hypotension secondary to guanethidine, or the rauwolfia-induced stuffy nose and thiazide-induced hypokalaemia and hyperuricaemia.

All of the antihypertensive drugs produce some side-effects; the most common of these are listed in Table 6. Before utilizing any therapeutic agent, the risk of its use must be balanced against the risk of the untreated disease and the benefits of treatment; a fundamental rule of therapeutics. Data are clear that the benefits derived from treating hypertension far outweigh the risk of side-effects of the available antihypertensive drugs[18]. Some of the more common side-effects that may limit the usefulness of specific drugs are listed below.

Table 5   Suggested dosages of commonly used antihypertensive drugs

	Diastolic pressure 90–114 mmHg		Diastolic pressure over 115 mmHg	
	Initial dose (mg/day)	Maximum dose (mg/day)	Initial dose (mg/day)	Maximum dose (mg/day)
Diuretics				
Hydrochlorothiazide	25–50	50–100	50	150
Chlorthalidone	25–50	50–100	50	100
Rauwolfia				
Whole root	50	100	50	100
Reserpine	0·1	0·25	0·25	0·25
Methyldopa	500	2000	750	2500
Propranolol*	40	320	160	480*
Hydralazine	50	250	75	300
Guanethidine	12·5	100	25	300
Clonidine	0·1	1·0	0·1	1·0–1·5
Prazosin	1·0	5·0–10·0	1·0	10·0–15·0

* Exact dosage limit not as yet determined.

NOTE: Diuretics, reserpine, and guanethidine can be given in single daily doses. Methyldopa, hydralazine, propranolol, prazosin, and clonidine should be given in two to four divided doses.

Rauwolfia drugs

Stuffy nose
This may be so annoying that patients may insist on stopping therapy. Antihistamines and nose-drops may relieve this symptom.

Change in mentation and/or depression
The occurrence of either of these side-effects is an indication to stop medication. The fear of such a reaction has led some physicians to eliminate the use of rauwolfia drugs; this despite the fact that they are as effective as other Step 2 agents, are less expensive, and are simple to use (one or at most two pills per day). We continue to obtain good results with rauwolfia drugs both in clinic and private practice settings. In patients with a history of depression or those undergoing emotional crises, etc., the drug should not be used. If nightmares or insomnia occur in a patient taking these drugs, drugs probably should be stopped. The original data possibly linking use of rauwolfia drugs with breast cancer[19] have been refuted by several different investigators[20].

Table 6 Side-effects of commonly used orally effective antihypertensive drugs

Drug	Trade name	Dosage (mg/day)	Side-effects
Diuretics			Serum chemistry abnormalities
Hydrochlorothiazide	Hydrodiuril Esidrix	50–100	↓potassium ↑uric acid
Chlorthalidone	Hygroton	50–100	↑urea nitrogen ↑blood glucose
			Blood dyscrasias, photosensitivity, gastrointestinal upsets, pancreatitis*
Rauwolfia derivatives			Sedation, bradycardia, nasal congestion, nightmares, depression, gastric ulcer
Reserpine	Serpasil	0·1–0·25	
Whole root	Raudixin	50–100	
Hydralazine	Apresoline	100–250	Headaches, tachycardia more if used alone. Rheumatoid-like syndrome, lupus reaction†
Guanethidine	Ismelin	10–150 or more	Weakness, diarrhoea, loss of ability to ejaculate orthostatic hypotension
Methyldopa	Aldomet	500–2500	Drowsiness, depression, oedema, impotence, abnormal liver function tests, fever, orthostatic hypotension, haemolytic anaemia, positive Coombs
Propranolol	Inderal	40–480	Insomnia, bradycardia, bronchospasm, heart failure, masking of insulin hypoglycaemia.
Clonidine	Catapres	0·1–1·5	Drowsiness, fatigue, dry mouth, 'Withdrawal hypertension'
Prazosin	Minipres	1·0–8–10·0	Syncope (early in treatment) Postural hypotension (occasionally)

* Many side-effects, for example blood dyscrasias and pancreatitis, are rare with diuretics.

† Rare with doses under 300 mg.

Diuretics

Concern on the part of some physicians about excess potassium loss with the use of diuretics, especially in elderly patients, often results in withholding these drugs from the treatment regimen and may account for the fact that only 2 years ago almost 25% of all initial prescriptions for newly discovered hypertensive patients were written for alpha-methyldopa, reserpine or propranolol rather than for diuretics. In our experience, *clinically significant* hypokalaemia is an unusual occurrence. Serum potassium levels decrease by an average of 0·5 mEq/l when measured in large numbers of patients taking diuretics (from approximately 4·2–4·4 mEq/l to 3·7–3·9 mEq/l). The average daily American diet contains approximately 60–100 mEq of potassium (2·3–3·9 g of potassium). Since the usual daily potassium requirement is only about one-half to one-third of this, or 20–50 mEq K^+ per day, there is a built-in 'excess intake', and a clinically significant deficiency is not produced in the majority of patients while they are taking diuretics.

In many patients, the addition of 20–25 mEq of potassium to their usual dietary intake at the time when diuretics are first started will suffice to prevent hypokalaemia. Serum levels of 3·5–4·0 mEq/1 are usually not an indication for supplemental therapy unless the patient is symptomatic (weakness, muscle cramps, etc.). If levels fall below 3·2 mEq/l, we are inclined to use potassium supplements or potassium-sparing drugs. The evidence available to date, however, indicates that the hypokalaemia associated with thiazide administration does not reflect a *major* deficit of total body potassium. The recent availability of total body counters has provided more reliable methods of measuring this deficit. Using this technique, several investigators have found that the fall in serum potassium with thiazide treatment is not accompanied by a significant change in total body potassium[21,22]. While there is some loss of potassium, particularly during the first 48 h, the total deficit over a period of approximately 1 month of continuous treatment represents only a small fraction of the total body potassium[23]. Such results suggest that thiazide-induced hypokalaemia represents a shift rather than a major loss of potassium from the body.

All patients who are taking *digitalis* should be started on potassium supplements or a potassium-sparing drug when diuretics are begun, to avoid possible digitalis toxicity. In elderly patients whose food intake may be limited, potassium supplements should also be used. Cost of foods with a high potassium content must be considered when advising a high potassium diet, especially in patients on limited incomes (Table 7). Our patients are given a list of foods that are high in potassium (Table 8) when therapy is started. This is included in the booklet, '*High Blood Pressure and What You Can Do About It*' (available from the Benjamin

Table 7 Foods or medications to provide approximately 40 mEq K⁺

Supplements	Quantity			Approximate cost (US cents)
Liquid	Kay Ciel		1 oz.	55
	Kaochlor	10%	1 oz.	48–50
	Generic KCl	10%	1 oz.	15–20
Tablets	Slow K – 5 tablets			40
Foods				
Orange juice	28 oz.	+ 350 calories		45–50
Bananas	22 oz.	+ 350 calories		30–35
Dried apricots	6 oz.	+ 450 calories		80–90

Table 8 Foods relatively high in potassium and low in sodium

Fruits	Vegetables
Apples, raw, whole	Asparagus, frozen
Apricots, canned, dried	Beans, white, cooked
Avocado	Beans, snap, green, cooked
Banana*	Brussels sprouts, fresh, frozen
Cantaloupe	Cabbage, shredded
Dates, dried, pitted	Cauliflower, fresh, frozen
Grapefruit	Corn on the cob
Nectarine, raw	Lima beans, fresh, cooked
Prunes, dried, cooked	Peas, green, cooked
Raisins, dried, seeded*	Peppers, green, raw
Watermelon	Potato, baked*
	Potato, boiled, no skin
Fruit juices	Radish, red, raw
Apple, fresh, canned	Squash, frozen, cooked
Grapefruit, canned	
Prune, canned	
Orange, fresh, canned frozen*	

* Especially helpful.

Extra amounts of the above foods will prevent a potassium deficiency.

Co., 485 Madison Ave, New York, NY).

Most liquid potassium supplements have a bitter taste. For this reason, we prefer to use Slow K tablets (one to four daily). These are safe, effective, and well-tolerated; each tablet contains 8 mEq of potassium.

There are several potassium-sparing drugs available. We prefer the use of triamterene for several reasons. Although this drug is not useful as a diuretic when utilized alone, it is an effective potassium-sparing agent when given with a thiazide diuretic (a combination capsule, Dyazide, is available). Usually one or two capsules a day are effective. Gastrointestinal side-effects may occur and, in patients with renal disease, hyperkalaemia is a potentially serious problem. Spironolactone, an aldosterone antagonist and another potassium-sparing drug, is a more effective diuretic than triamterene when used alone, but is generally also given with a thiazide in a combination pill, aldactoside. Two to four pills a day must be given; it is more expensive, and side-effects, especially gynaecomastia, are more annoying. As noted, in the majority of patients, diuretics can be given without the use of supplements or sparing drugs.

The fear of causing or aggravating *hyperuricaemia* is another deterrent to the use of diuretics. This often leads to improper or inadequate therapy, as was noted in a 58-year-old man who was being treated with many different drugs for three years with little or no blood pressure response (Figure 1). Only token diuretic therapy was being given because of a pre-treatment uric acid elevation (11·2 mg%). In 1972 he was finally treated adequately with appropriate diuretics, and has been maintained at normal blood pressure levels since that time. He did develop gout and now requires Allopurinol to control uric acid levels; his prognosis has been greatly improved by treatment.

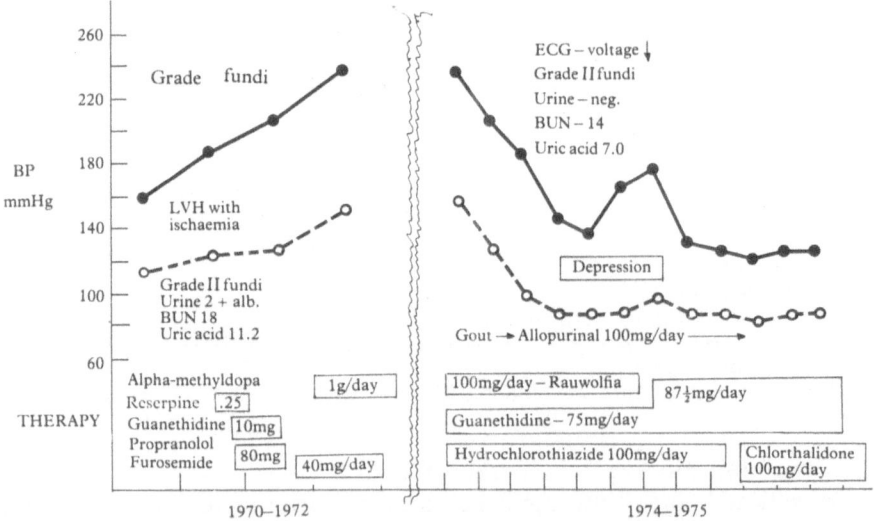

Figure 1 58-year-old male; hypertension of 5 years duration. Poor blood pressure response until adequate dosages of diuretics and guanethidine were used. Diuretics initially withheld in full doses because of high serum uric levels. Reprinted from Moser, M. (1977). Long-term management of hypertension. *N.Y. State J. Med.*, 77, 76

Although gout can be annoying, and a rising uric acid level a concern, these side-effects can be managed and should not mitigate against using diuretic drugs if they are needed to control blood pressure; the risk is outweighed by the benefit of therapy. A new diuretic, ticrynafen, that is an effective antihypertensive drug and also lowers uric acid levels, is presently under investigation.

Propranolol
Insomnia and dreams are frequent side-effects. These sometimes persist, regardless of timing of the dosage. Precipitation of asthmatic attacks in susceptible individuals is also a major problem. Some of the newer beta-blockers (not as yet approved for use in the United States) are cardio-selective and are said to cause less bronchospasm. Beta-blockers are contraindicated in the presence of congestive heart failure.

Alpha-methyldopa
Fatigue, drowsiness and depression can be quite prominent side-effects with this drug.

Clonidine
Dry mouth and drowsiness are frequent side-effects; some patients will flatly refuse to continue taking clonidine because of this. Abrupt withdrawal of clonidine may result in a serious hypertensive reaction.

Prazosin
A severe hypotensive (syncopal) reaction occasionally occurs after the first dose of this drug.

Impotence
Impotence can be an annoying side-effect of almost all of the antihypertensive drugs. With some, such as guanethidine, erection and intercourse is possible; normal ejaculation is inhibited; with other drugs, such as reserpine or alpha-methyldopa, erection is inhibited or incomplete. This is an extremely difficult problem to manage, especially when it occurs in young men who have significant hypertension, where treatment is extremely important. Some patients may have to be convinced to tolerate this 'side-effect', at least until blood pressure lowering is accomplished. At that time, changing medication and trying different combinations, such as a diuretic with propranolol, may be helpful in restoring potency. We have been successful in managing this problem in some instances by omitting one or several drugs for a day or two each week, once blood pressure control has been achieved. Impotence is by no means a universal side-effect of antihypertensive drugs, and when it occurs in older men, may actually represent a non-drug-related phenomenon. The incidence of this annoying side-effect varies greatly in different reported series.

HOME BLOOD PRESSURES

Home blood pressure recordings have been advocated by many investigators as an aid and an incentive to the patient in understanding the process of treatment, and as an aid to the physician in adjusting dosages of medication. While we believe that home blood pressure recordings may be helpful in a small percentage of patients who are receiving multiple and potent drugs, or who might be engaged in an occupation that requires frequent postural changes, we do not believe that this procedure should be routine in the majority of hypertensive patients. Excellent long-term blood pressure control has been achieved in over 80% of our patients without the use of this technique[24]. We believe that, in many instances, it contributes to anxiety and makes the family and the patient over-conscious of the blood pressure 'problem'. One goal of the treatment programme of a chronic disease, such as hypertension, is to prevent the patient from becoming over-tense or neurotic about his or her disease. Home blood pressures may be of use during the initial stages of drug adjustment, especially where potent agents, such as guanethidine, are to be used, or in some patients who might be quite insistent upon knowing their exact pressure readings. However, in our experience, we have not found this procedure necessary in order to obtain good treatment results.

There are many investigators who feel quite differently about the use of home blood pressure recordings. In their experience, the repeated taking of pressures seems to reduce anxiety and increase the patient's adherence to the treatment programme.

SPECIAL PROBLEMS: HIGH BLOOD PRESSURE IN THE ELDERLY

Blood pressure lowering in elderly patients presents a special problem. Although the added risk of both systolic and diastolic pressure elevations is well-documented in this group, data are not available that define benefits of reducing pressure to normal levels, i.e., 140/90 mmHg. Benefit may not be greater than risk in some cases. In addition, many older patients react poorly to antihypertensive drugs. Cerebral vessel autoregulation is decreased, renal function significantly less, and cardiac reserve diminished as compared to younger patients. Sudden changes in blood pressure may produce annoying or even dangerous symptoms[25].

Despite the lack of data, we believe that elevated pressure in patients over 65 years of age should be lowered, *if* this can be accomplished by a simple regimen without significant side-effects. The use of diuretics, propranolol or in fact any of the effective antihypertensive agents, is acceptable if careful attention is paid to titrating drug dosages slowly. Unfortunately, a definite percentage (approximately 25% in our series) of these patients will not be successfully treated to normotensive levels because of intolerable side-effects.

SUMMARY

The following points are of importance in treating patients with essential hypertension.

(a) Once a definite diagnosis of hypertension is made, i.e. over 140/90 mmHg in patients 50 years or younger and over 160/95 mmHg in older patients, therapy should be pursued to a goal of normotensive levels (below 140/90 mmHg) if at all possible.

(b) In patients with diastolic pressures below 105 mmHg, methods other than specific drugs can be tried; unfortunately they are often ineffective. If other risk factors for cardiovascular disease are also present, therapy with antihypertensive medications is clearly indicated.

(c) The stepped-care approach, while empiric, is effective in a high percentage of cases. Diuretics should be used as the first drug in almost all cases. Medications should be added or substituted until goal blood pressure is achieved.

(e) If the physician is motivated and convinced that therapy is useful, he can usually motivate his patient. Successful blood pressure lowering can be achieved in over 80% of patients over long periods of time.

References

1 Kannel, W. B., McGee, D. and Gordon, T. (1976). A general cardiovascular risk profile: the Framingham Study. *Am. J. Cardiol.*, **38**, 46

2 Moser, M. (1977). The prognosis of effectively treated hypertension. In G. Onesti and D. T. Lowenthal (eds.). *The Spectrum of Antihypertensive Drug Therapy*, pp. 1–10. (New York: Biomedical Information Corporation)

3 Julius, S. and Schork, M. A. (1971). Borderline hypertension: a critical review. *J. Chronic. Dis.* **23**, 723

4 Report of the Joint National Committee on Detection, Evaluation and Treatment of High Blood Pressure (1977). *J. Am. Med. Assoc.*, **237**, 225

5 Tucker, R. M. and Labarthe, D. R. (1977). Frequency of surgical treatment for hypertension in adults at the Mayo Clinic from 1973 through 1975. *Mayo Clin. Proc.*, **52**, 549

6 Kempner, W. (1948). Treatment of hypertensive vascular disease with rice diet. *Am. J. Med.* **4**, 545

7 Parijs, J., Joosens, J. V., Van der Linden, L., *et al.* (1973). Moderate sodium restriction and diuretics in the treatment of hypertension. *Am. Heart J.*, **85**, 22

8 Moser, M. (1959). The effect of a high salt diet on the treatment of essential hypertension. In J. H. Moyer (ed.). *Hahnemann Symposium on Hypertension*, p. 512. (Philadelphia: Saunders)

9 Moser, M. and Goldman, A. G. (1967). *Hypertensive Vascular Disease.* (Philadelphia: J. B. Lippincott)

10 Chiang, N., Perlman, L. V. and Epstein, F. H. (1969). Overweight and hypertension. *Circulation*, **39**, 403

11 Wallace, R. K. (1970). Physiological effects of transcendental meditation. *Science*, **167**, 1751

12 Shapiro, A. P. *et al.* (1977). Behavioral methods in the treatment of hypertension. *Ann. Intern. Med.*, **86**, 626

13 Gordon, T., Kannel, W. B., Dawber, T. R. and McGee, D. (1975). Changes associated with quitting cigarette smoking: the Framingham Study. *Am. Heart J.*, **90**, 322

14 Cooper, E. H. and Cranston, W. I. (1957). A comparison of the effects of phenobarbitone and reserpine in hypertension. *Lancet*, **1**, 396

15 Krogsgaard, A. R. (1957). Hypotensive effect of reserpine compared with phenobarbital and placebo. *Acta Med. Scand.*, **157**, 379

16 Moser, M. (1977). Physician adherence in the management of hypertension. (In press) abst – *Prev. Med.*, Mar. 1978.

17 Veterans Administration Cooperative Study Group on Antihypertensive Agents (1977). Propranolol in the treatment of essential hypertension. *J. Am. Med. Assoc.*, **237**, 2303

18 Veterans Administration Cooperative Study Group on Antihypertensive Agents (1967). Effects of treatment on morbidity in hypertension. Results in patients with diastolic blood pressures averaging 115 through 129 mmHg. *J. Am. Med. Assoc.*, **202**, 1028

19 Boston Collaborative Drug Surveillance Program (1974). Reserpine and breast cancer. *Lancet*, **2**, 669

20 O'Fallon, W. M., Labarthe, D. R. and Kurland, L. T. (1975). Rauwolfia derivatives and breast cancer. *Lancet*, **2**, 292

21 Graybiel, L. G. and Sode, J. (1971). Diuretics, potassium depletion and carbohydrate intolerance. *Lancet*, **2**, 265

22 Wilkinson, P. R. and Issler, H. (1975). Total body and serum potassium during prolonged thiazide therapy for essential hypertension. *Lancet*, **1**, 759

23 Maronde, R. F., Milgiom, M. and Dickey, J. M. (1969). Potassium loss with thiazide therapy. *Am. Heart J.*, **78**, 16

24 Moser, M. (1974). Office management of hypertension. *Am. Fam. Physician*, **10**, 152

25 Chrysant, S. G., Frohlich, E. D. and Papper, S. (1976). Why hypertension is so prevalent in the elderly – and how to treat it. *Geriatrics*, **31**, 101

6

Treatment of special forms of hypertension

M. D. Guazzi

Hypertensive crisis

INTRODUCTION

Hypertension is usually treated by appropriate orally administered antihypertensive agents, and several weeks of observation are generally required for satisfactory titration of dosage against pressure response and side-effects of the drugs. On occasion, however, blood pressure rises so precipitously and severely, or the clinical condition in which hypertension occurs is so critical, that prompt pressure lowering becomes crucial to prevent disabling, or even lethal, complications.

These crisis situations (Table 1) may take origin from several clinical disorders. They develop rarely in previously normotensive persons

Table 1   Hypertensive emergencies*

Malignant hypertension

Acute hypertensive encephalopathy

Severe hypertension associated with acute or chronic glomerulonephritis

Hypertension complicated by:
  Intracerebral or subarachnoid haemorrhage
  Acute left ventricular failure
  Acute aortic dissection

Hypertension with or without bleeding in the postoperative period of cardiac and vascular reparative surgery

Hypertensive crisis of phaeochromocytoma, drug and food interaction with MAO inhibitors, clonidine withdrawal

* Eclampsia is discussed elsewhere.

115

during the course of acute glomerulonephritis, eclampsia, collagen disease or head injury; more commonly they complicate the accelerated phase of untreated or poorly treated chronic hypertension of various aetiologies. Their prominent characteristics are necrotizing arteriolitis; spasm of arterioles; organ damage, such as cardiac failure, renal failure, encephalopathy or neuroretinitis. Phaeochromocytoma, or the release of tissue catecholamines by certain drugs or foods in patients during monoamine oxidase (MAO) inhibitor therapy, represent other causes of abrupt pressure elevation.

There is also a group of conditions that qualify as hypertensive emergencies not so much because of the actual height of the pressure, but rather because of complicating disorders that make even moderate pressure elevation harmful. These include acute aortic dissection, intracranial bleeding and acute left ventricular failure.

Two fundamental concepts in the management of hypertensive emergencies are as follows:

(1). Immediate and intense therapy is required and takes precedence over time-consuming diagnostic procedures; because of the rapid progress of vascular damage the degree of reversibility of complications will depend on the speed with which effective treatment is instituted.

(2) The choice of drugs will depend on how their time course of action and their haemodynamic and metabolic effects meet the needs of the crisis situation.

Therefore, no single antihypertensive agent should always be selected as the first choice for treating a hypertensive crisis.

DRUG THERAPY

The pharmacological and therapeutic attributes of the drugs currently used to reduce arterial pressure in hypertensive emergencies are listed in Tables 2 and 3. A guide for their prime indications and contraindications is provided in Table 4. A list of new drugs that might find their place in the therapeutic armamentarium of the hypertensive crisis is shown at the end of this chapter.

Diazoxide
Diazoxide is chemically related to the thiazide diuretics. This potent and rapidly effective antihypertensive drug was introduced in the market for intravenous treatment of hypertensive emergencies. It causes a prompt and usually considerable fall of systolic and diastolic pressure which is

Table 2 Drugs for treatment of hypertensive emergencies: route of administration, dosage, time course of action

Drug	Route of administration and dosage			Time course of action		
	Intra-muscular (mg)	Intra-venous (mg)	Inter-val (h)	Onset	Peak	Duration
Diazoxide (Hyperstat)	—	100–600	4–5	3–5 min	2–3 h	4–18 h
Hydralazine (Apresoline)	10–30	10–30	3–6	10–30 min	20–40 min	3–8 h
Methyldopa (Aldomet)	—	300–600	4–8	1–3 h	3–5 h	6–12 h
Pentolinium tartrate (Ansolysen)	2–20	—	4–5	15–30 min		5–6 h
Phentolamine mesylate (Regitine)	10–20	5–10		1–3 min	3–5 min	5–10 min
Reserpine	0·5–5	0·5–5	4–12	1–3 h	3–6 h	6–24 h
	Intravenous infusion (mg/min)					
Sodium nitro-prusside (Nipride)	0·03–0·5			1/2–1 min	1–2 min	2–4 min
Trimethaphan camsylate (Arfonad)	1–15			2–5 min	3–7 min	7–10 min

entirely due to a reduction of vascular resistance through vascular smooth muscle relaxation. This effect, which involves in greater degree the resistance vessels[1–3], and to a minimal extent the capacitance ones[4], seems to be due to a calcium antagonistic action[5]. Increase in heart-rate, stroke volume, velocity of ventricular ejection and cardiac output associated with the pressure decrease, is due to a reflex sympathetic outflow elicited by baroreceptor activation[1,2,4,6–8]. Heart-rate and cardiac output increments tend to raise the work of the heart, and might be detrimental to patients with reduced coronary or cardiac reserve. This effect, however, has not been an important problem during the clinical use of this agent. It is conceivable that the beneficial influence exerted by the decreased pressure load and, hence, myocardial wall stress during ejection, is such as to overcome the negative effect of

Table 3 Drugs for treatment of hypertensive emergencies: mechanism of action, haemodynamic responses and side-effects

Drug	Mechanism of action	Haemodynamic responses				Side-effects
		HR	CO	TPR	Contractility	
Diazoxide	Direct dilatation of arterioles	↑	↑	↓	↑	Hyperglycaemia, nausea, vomiting, tachycardia, chest pain, fluid retention, postural hypotension, extrapyramidal symptoms
Hydralazine	Direct dilatation of arterioles	↑	↑	↓	↑	Tachycardia, aggravation of angina, headache, flushing, nausea, fluid retention
Methyldopa	Decreased sympathetic vaso-motor stimulation. Direct dilatation of arterioles (?)	↓	↑↓	↑↓	↓	Somnolence
Pentolinium tartrate	Ganglionic blockade	↑	↑↓	↓	↓	Postural hypotension, dry mouth, paresis of bowel and bladder
Phentolamine mesylate	Arteriolar dilatation through alpha-adrenergic receptors blockade and direct action	↑	↑	↓	—	Tachycardia, nausea, serious or even fatal hypotension
Reserpine	Decreased sympathetic vasomotor stimulation	↑	—	↓	↓	Activation of peptic ulcer, stupor, somnolence
Sodium nitroprusside	Direct dilatation of arterioles and veins	↑	↓	↓	—	Thiocyanate intoxication, muscular twitching, vomiting, agitation
Trimethaphan camsylate	Ganglionic blockade	↑	↑↓	↓	↓	Postural hypotension, dry mouth

Table 4   Drugs for treatment of hypertensive emergencies: indications and contraindications

Drug	Indications	Contraindications or use with caution
Diazoxide	Malignant hypertension Acute hypertensive encephalopathy Postoperative period (?) Acute left ventricular failure	Intracranial haemorrhage Coronary insufficiency Acute aortic dissection Diabetes Postoperative bleeding
Hydralazine	Same as diazoxide	Acute left ventricular failure Acute aortic dissection Coronary insufficiency
Methyldopa	Postoperative period	Acute hypertensive encephalopathy Intracranial haemorrhage
Pentolinium tartrate	Malignant hypertension Acute hypertensive encephalopathy Acute left ventricular failure	Postoperative period Renal insufficiency
Phentolamine mesylate	Hypertensive crisis of phaeochromocytoma, during MAO inhibitors therapy or clonidine withdrawal	Severe hypertension associated with volume depletion
Reserpine	Malignant hypertension Postoperative period Acute aortic dissection	Acute hypertensive encephalopathy Intracranial haemorrhage Peptic ulcer
Sodium nitroprusside	Acute hypertensive encephalopathy Hypertensive crisis during MAO inhibitors therapy Acute left ventricular failure Intracranial haemorrhage Postoperative period	
Trimethaphan camsylate	Acute left ventricular failure Intracranial haemorrhage Acute aortic dissection	Postoperative period Renal insufficiency

tachycardia and increased volume load[9]. This probably represents the rational basis for the confident use of the drug to reduce blood pressure in patients presenting with left ventricular failure[10]. Since cardiovascular reflexes and sympathetic nervous system function are not impaired, severe postural hypotension is an uncommon side-effect[7,11]. Nevertheless, a 10° head-up tilt may potentiate the hypotensive response to diazoxide, and has been suggested as a useful adjunct in poorly responding cases[12].

Diazoxide causes retention of sodium and water and expansion of plasma volume; frank oedema formation is the rule in patients with myocardial inadequacy[14]. These effects can readily be antagonized by furosemide or ethacrynic acid. Increased concentration of free fatty acids, hyperuricaemia and hyperglycaemia do not represent major problems, but preclude use of the drug for long-term treatment of hypertension. Cardiac arrhythmias, palpitation, headache and flushing are occasionally observed after diazoxide; occurrence of anginal pain[15], of disabling cerebral and cardiac complications[16] has been reported.

Diazoxide has become an agent of choice for most hypertensive emergencies; it is unique, among the agents currently used in these disorders, in lowering arterial pressure towards, or to, normal; both promptly and for several hours. The ordinary intravenous dose is 300 mg or 5 mg/kg. To achieve the best effect the full dose should be injected quite rapidly, within 10–30 s, in view of the fact that diazoxide is 90% bound to plasma albumin. A distinct advantage is that constant patient monitoring is not required. The major disadvantage is that the fall in blood pressure cannot be titrated; abrupt reductions can be hazardous in atherosclerotic patients with coronary and cerebral impairment, although such complications are surprisingly rare.

Diazoxide and other agents which directly reduce vascular smooth muscle tone are not advised in the presence of intracranial or postoperative bleeding. Finally, the increase in stroke output and velocity of ventricular ejection contraindicates the drug for pressure reduction in cases of acute aortic dissection.

Hydralazine
Adequate doses of hydralazine decrease diastolic and systolic blood pressure and peripheral vascular resistance, and increase heart-rate and stroke volume. Present evidence indicates that its major action is direct relaxation of vascular smooth muscle; the effect is greater on arterioles than on veins. Cardiac stimulation probably involves a reflex sympathetic response to the fall in blood pressure, as well as direct effect on the heart. The peripheral vasodilatation, which develops gradually over 15–30 min after intravenous administration, is widespread. Cerebral and renal blood flow increase unless the fall in blood pressure is very profound. Glomerular filtration rate and renal tubular function are not consistently influenced; however, like many other vasodilators, hydralazine can produce sodium retention, urinary volume reduction, and increase in renin secretion. The hyperdynamic circulation induced by this agent may accentuate specific disorders related to cardiac and

coronary insufficiency.

In approximately 10% of cases receiving high doses (in excess of 400 mg daily) there is the occurrence of an acute rheumatoid state, and in a smaller percentage a syndrome resembling disseminated lupus erythematosus. A possible immunological mechanism for these reactions has been postulated[17]. These symptoms usually remit with discontinuance of the drug.

Although this compound is most commonly used in its oral form for patients with less severe hypertension, it is a potent antihypertensive when administered parenterally. After intravenous injection of 10–30 mg, blood pressure will fall within 30–40 min. The injection must be repeated every 3–8 h. This agent is especially suited for hypertensive emergencies associated with renal insufficiency as the decrease of blood pressure is usually not accompanied by a proportional decrease in renal blood flow. Coronary insufficiency, acute left ventricular failure, and aortic dissection represent its major contraindications.

Methyldopa
Since 1960, when its hypotensive properties were noted[18], methyldopa has come to be one of the major agents used in the treatment of high blood pressure. It causes progressive reduction in blood pressure and heart-rate, which is maximal at 3–8 h, and may persist for as long as 24 h. Even after intravenous administration the hypertensive effect is not apparent for at least 1–3 h.

The fall in blood pressure has been variously reported to be due to decrease in cardiac output, peripheral vascular resistance, or both[19]. Present evidence suggests that the major antihypertensive effect of methyldopa is due to an action on the central nervous system; some contribution of peripheral mechanisms, however, cannot be excluded. Although blood pressure may be somewhat lower in the orthostatic than in the supine position, symptomatic orthostatic hypotension is uncommon. The reduction in blood pressure following methyldopa has not been shown to involve any major changes in blood flow distribution; glomerular filtration rate and renal blood flow are maintained or increased in hypertensive patients with both normal and impaired renal function. The drug decreases plasma renin activity, but still tends to cause sodium and water retention. Given orally or parenterally it causes sedation which tends to decrease with continued treatment. The hypotensive response to 500–1000 mg administered intravenously may be variable: in some patients there is little or no effect, and even paradoxical hypertension may occur.

Because of its delayed onset of action, it is more useful in hypertensive crises that do not require hypotension within moments. Its advantage is that once the antihypertensive effect is achieved (possibly in association with diuretics), oral treatment may be instituted without need for introducing another preparation. It may cause sufficient drowsiness to interfere with the neurological evaluation in hypertensive encephalopathy or intracranial bleeding. Methyldopa may find its best indication in the management of accelerated hypertension associated with acute or chronic renal parenchymal disease.

Pentolinium tartrate and trimethaphan camsylate

These agents are ganglion-blocking drugs. Following ganglionic blockade blood pressure may be decreased only minimally in the recumbent position, but may fall markedly when the patient is sitting or standing. Elevation of the head of the bed is utilized in clinical practice to potentiate the hypotensive effects of these drugs. In subjects undergoing this therapy, total peripheral resistance is decreased, the output of the normal heart is often reduced (probably as a consequence of a diminished venous return resulting from venous dilatation and peripheral pooling of blood), while the output of the failing heart is frequently increased (due to a reduction of cardiac filling pressure and impedance to ejection). Renal effects include a decrease of glomerular filtration rate and renal blood flow, and an increase in renal vascular resistance.

Trimethaphan is extremely short-acting and can be given only by continuous intravenous infusion for controlled hypotension or for emergency treatment of hypertensive crises; the rate of infusion is adjusted to maintain the desired level of blood pressure. Because it reduces myocardial contractility and, hence, ejection velocity, trimethaphan is a useful drug in the treatment of aortic dissection. The need for close blood pressure monitoring and for expert personnel cannot be overemphasized. Pentolinium is given by intramuscular injection, and constant monitoring is not essential.

Due to parasympathetic, as well as sympathetic, blockade the tone and motility of the gastrointestinal tract are reduced by these agents, and propulsion of the small intestine may be completely arrested; they also cause impairment of the voiding contractions of the urinary bladder. If the hypotension is excessive, anginal attacks may be precipitated in patients with coronary insufficiency.

Ganglion-blocking drugs are suited for treating hypertensive crisis associated with elevated central venous pressure and congestive heart failure, but constant attention must be devoted to signs of paralytic ileus and urinary retention. When renal or coronary insufficiency complicate hypertension the use of other agents is preferable.

Reserpine

Despite the competition of newer drugs, reserpine still has its advocates. It suffers from the fact that onset of the antihypertensive action is delayed, and that the effective dose varies widely from one patient to another. It is a poor choice when a true emergency exists. In parenteral large doses it causes drowsiness which is undesirable in hypertensive encephalopathy, intracranial bleeding and head injury. Other important side-effects include depressive reactions, peptic ulcer formation and, occasionally, frank psychosis.

Phentolamine

This alpha-receptor blocker was introduced and in the past was used as a screening test for phaeochromocytoma. It has a specific place in the therapeutic management of phaeochromocytoma, in aborting harmful rises of blood pressure occurring during provocative tests, or during surgical removal of the tumour. It also can be used to treat the hypertensive rebound that may occur during withdrawal of clonidine, or in treating the hypertensive crisis secondary to release of tissue catecholamine that may occur in patients receiving MAO inhibitors. The hypotensive effect of a single intravenous bolus of phentolamine usually lasts less than 15 min; intravenous infusion is consequently desirable after the blood pressure has been controlled by the intravenous injection. Serious hypotension[20–22] may occur following phentolamine administered for diagnostic or therapeutic purposes in subjects with or without phaeochromocytoma. Cases have been reported of patients suffering from essential hypertension who developed shock following phentolamine injection[23]. Haemodynamic studies of these patients, an example of which is shown in Figure 1, usually reveal extreme vasoconstriction, hypovolaemia and low cardiac output. Because of such precarious states of circulatory adjustment a minimal stress, such as the vasodilatation induced by phentolamine, can induce severe hypotension[24]. The drug therefore must be administered with caution, and not to dehydrated patients with low extracellular and plasma volumes who are compensating by sympathetic stimulation and resulting vasoconstriction.

Sodium nitroprusside

This is an old drug of predictable and safe effectiveness even in refractory cases. In the past it has been largely neglected because of its instability, and because it has not been commercially available for intravenous use. It has recently become commercially available and nitroprusside is becoming a strong contender as the drug of choice in a large number of hypertensive emergencies. It must be given by intravenous infusion under continuous monitoring of the blood pressure response. The blood

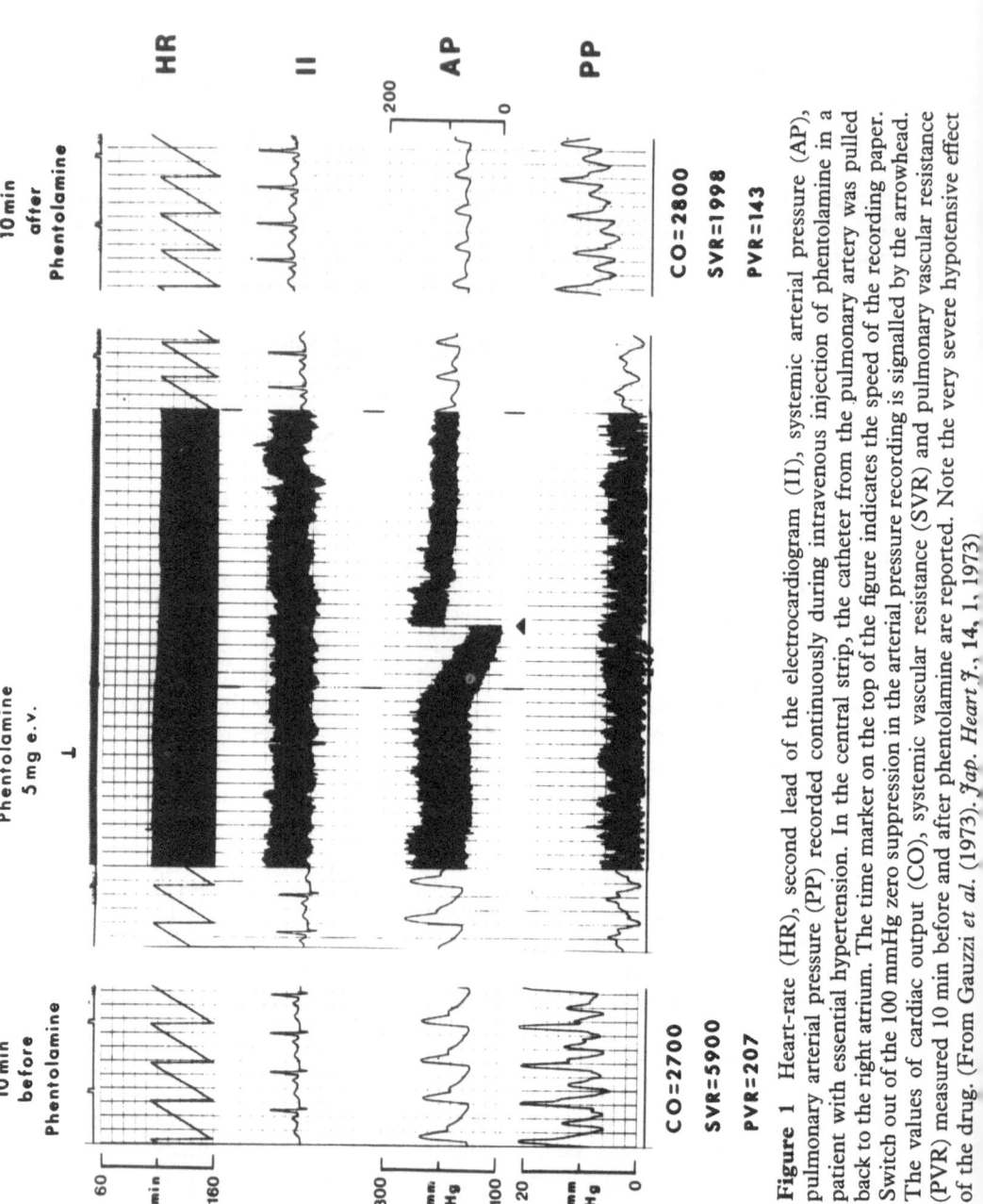

Figure 1 Heart-rate (HR), second lead of the electrocardiogram (II), systemic arterial pressure (AP), pulmonary arterial pressure (PP) recorded continuously during intravenous injection of phentolamine in a patient with essential hypertension. In the central strip, the catheter from the pulmonary artery was pulled back to the right atrium. The time marker on the top of the figure indicates the speed of the recording paper. Switch out of the 100 mmHg zero suppression in the arterial pressure recording is signalled by the arrowhead. The values of cardiac output (CO), systemic vascular resistance (SVR) and pulmonary vascular resistance (PVR) measured 10 min before and after phentolamine are reported. Note the very severe hypotensive effect of the drug. (From Gauzzi *et al.* (1973), *Jap. Heart J.*, **14**, 1, 1973)

pressure can be maintained at almost any level by adjusting the infusion rate. Undesirable hypotension is treated simply by temporary discontinuance of the infusion, since the duration of its effect is evanescent.

The hypotensive response to nitroprusside, which is potentiated by head-up tilting, is due to relaxation of arteriolar and venular smooth muscle[8]. The fall in pressure is associated with a reduced total peripheral resistance, small changes in cardiac output, some increase in heart-rate. Because it reduces pre-load and impedance to left ventricular ejection, not only will this drug immediately diminish pressure and remit symptoms in hypertensive encephalopathy, but it is also beneficial to patients with angina pectoris, myocardial infarction, refractory heart failure of various aetiologies, with or without hypertension[25,26]. Hypertensive emergencies associated with aortic dissection, intracranial haemorrhage or cardiovascular reconstructive procedures, represent other indications for the use of nitroprusside. In aortic dissection it probably should be administered in association with a beta-adrenergic blocking drug.

Prolonged administration, especially to patients with renal insufficiency, can result in thiocyanate toxicity[27] which is formed during metabolic degradation of nitroprusside.

CONDITIONS ASSOCIATED WITH HYPERTENSIVE CRISIS

Malignant hypertension

Patients with severe accelerated (malignant) hypertension must be considered medical emergencies[29]. Malignant hypertension ordinarily manifests itself by greatly elevated diastolic pressure, rapidly progressive symptoms and signs at the level of the central nervous system (from headache to convulsions and coma), retina (blurring vision, exudates, haemorrhages, papilloedema, severe arteriolar constriction), kidney (proteinuria, haematuria, cylindruria and azotaemia), and heart (occult or overt cardiac insufficiency). It can result from primary hypertension, hypertension secondary to renal vascular or parenchymal diseases, or phaeochromocytoma.

Evidence is convincing that it is not so much the underlying cause for hypertension as it is the blood pressure *per se* which sustains the malignant phase and causes the complications. Consequently patients manifesting severe accelerated hypertension should be hospitalized at once, preferentially in an intensive-care unit. Treatment should be started promptly with the aim of reducing blood pressure within a few hours to a few days. Diagnostic procedures, other than serum electrolytes and crea-

tinine, urinalysis, haemogram, chest X-ray and ECG, should not interfere with the promptness of institution of treatment. With the exception
of phaeochromocytoma the choice among the agents listed on Table 2
and the need for drug combinations, such as diuretics plus beta-blockers,
depend almost exclusively on the severity of hypertension, presence and
types of complications. Treatment can begin on admission to the hospital
with diazoxide 300 mg intravenously, or hydralazine 15 mg. It is also
advisable to promote rapid diuresis with intravenous furosemide
80–160 mg, the larger dose being required in the presence of renal failure. Injections of diazoxide or hydralazine can be repeated as needed,
remembering that following the diuretic the response to the vasodilator
drugs will be enhanced. Once the blood pressure has been controlled, a
detailed diagnostic evaluation is needed and treatment is continued on
oral medications such as diuretic plus methyldopa, or a beta-adrenergic
blocker plus, if necessary, a vasodilator drug, such as hydralazine or prazosin. Doses and combinations must be such as to keep and maintain the
blood pressure as near to normal as possible. Prompt control of the blood
pressure will effectively prevent or reverse such serious and frequent
complications of malignant hypertension as left ventricular failure and
hypertensive encephalopathy.

Acute left ventricular failure
The functional response of the failing left ventricle to a reduced pressure
load is generally so favourable that resort to digitalis is often unnecessary. It follows that even modest hypertension should be treated
promptly with rapidly acting agents when pulmonary oedema is present.
Under these circumstances the ideal drug is the one which would reduce
the pre-load (venous return) as well as decrease the after-load (wall
stress during ejection and consequently metabolic need of the myocardium). The drug should not promote salt and water retention or reflex
tachycardia. Nitroprusside is the compound that more closely approaches the ideal drug[25–28]. Furosemide, in doses of 40–160 mg,
should be administered orally or intravenously, along with sodium nitroprusside. The ganglion-blocking agents are satisfactory alternatives to
this drug. Diazoxide may also be useful; in view of its prominent sodium
and water retention, the association of loop diuretics becomes even more
important.

Hypertensive encephalopathy
The severity of this complication is such that control of arterial pressure
within minutes to hours is mandatory. Headache, nausea, vomiting, apprehension and mental confusion, characterize the clinical picture. Neurological signs that may present include focal twitching, aphasia, vision

disturbances and positive Babinski sign. All these manifestations, which develop within hours to 1–2 days, are likely to progress to convulsions, coma and death if appropriate treatment is not instituted at once. The blood pressure is severely elevated with diastolic levels above 130 mmHg. The differential diagnosis of hypertensive encephalopathy involves other types of cerebrovascular accidents associated with hypertension: thrombosis, subarachnoid or intracerebral haemorrhage, and infarction with secondary hypertension.

It is desirable to have the patient admitted to an intensive-care unit, where blood pressure can be monitored and consciousness and patency of the airways inspected. Sodium nitroprusside is the drug of choice, the infusion rate being adjusted to maintain blood pressure at normal levels. When, for some reason, constant monitoring of blood pressure is not feasible, diazoxide in association with intravenous furosemide is preferable. Drugs such as reserpine and methyldopa, which may aggravate somnolence and interfere with the evaluation of consciousness level, should be avoided. Parenteral preparations should be maintained until oral treatment has been titrated to effective doses. For the latter, combinations of a diuretic plus an adrenergic blocking drug generally are used; if necessary a vasodilator drug is added.

SPECIAL THERAPEUTIC CONSIDERATIONS

Bleeding
Most authorities agree that intracerebral haemorrhage requires rapid reduction of arterial pressure to normal or even hypotensive levels. However, the patient must be closely watched to make sure that vital functions are not interfered with by the pressure reduction. Postoperative bleeding in the presence of severe hypertension also benefits from prompt pressure lowering. Direct arteriolar dilating agents should be avoided in this situation.

Renal failure
When hypertensive emergency is associated with renal failure, the necessity for treating blood pressure must be balanced against the risk of making the renal function worse. An over-cautious approach, however, is not justified in view of these arguments: uncontrolled hypertension increases renal damage, which in turn potentiates hypertension; reduction of blood pressure in patients with malignant hypertension complicated by renal insufficiency does not necessarily result in deterioration of renal function and may prolong survival[30,31]. The increase in serum creatinine or BUN which almost regularly occurs in the presence of renal fail-

ure is the result of a haemodynamic rather than a pathological effect. In the normal kidney glomerular filtration rate falls only briefly following antihypertensive agents, due to autonomous readjustments of the renal vessels. In the diseased kidney these vascular readjustments occur very slowly over several weeks. Thus, the worsening of the nitrogen usually is only temporary and subsides over a period of weeks if the blood pressure is controlled.

Care should be taken to choose antihypertensive drugs interfering as little as possible with renal blood flow. Diazoxide, hydralazine, sodium nitroprusside, methyldopa or minoxidil[32] are the drugs of choice. However, reduction in extracellular volume must also be induced, either by loop diuretics or by haemodialysis.

Coronary artery disease
Drastic reduction of arterial pressure in patients with impairment of coronary circulation should be avoided. The risk of producing myocardial infarction is minimized when arterial pressure is reduced gradually, with drugs such as diuretics and beta-adrenergic blocking agents, in combination if needed.

NEW DRUGS

Recently, drugs have been developed which block both beta- and alpha-adrenoreceptors[33,34]. Evidence is accumulating that they effectively lower blood pressure in hypertensive subjects[35]. When used intravenously they induce, within 10 min, a significant decrease of systolic and diastolic pressure through a predominant reduction of systemic vascular resistance[36]. Effectiveness in hypertensive crisis of phaeochromocytoma has also been reported[37].

Another group of drugs which deserves mention in this setting is the calcium antagonists, such as nifedipine. This drug reduces the oxygen consumption of the heart and induces vasodilatation through a depression of excitation–contraction coupling. These pharmacological properties have suggested the use of this compound in the therapy of ischaemic heart disease[38]. The relaxant action on the arterial smooth muscle (an angiographic documentation of this effect is reported in Figure 2) is such as to lower blood pressure in hypertension. In severe hypertension pressure reduction following 10 mg nifedipine is prompt, occurring within 5–15 min by the sublingual route, and considerable 24·3% decrease of mean arterial pressure from control[39]. The hypotensive response, which is exclusively due to peripheral vascular resistance reduction (heart-rate and stroke volume augment) persists for 2–3 h.

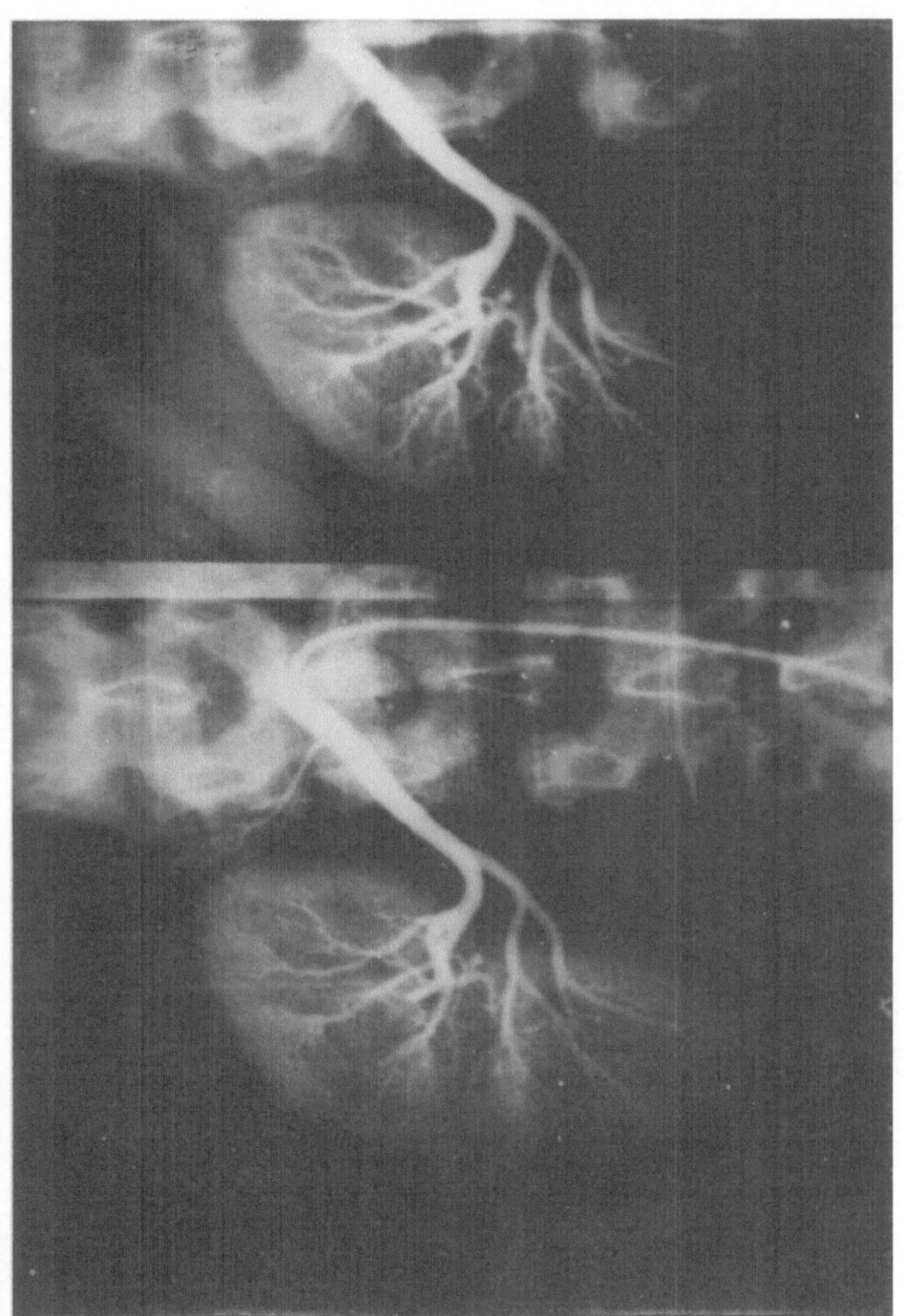

Figure 2 Renal arteriogram in a hypertensive subject, before (left) and 30 min after (right) oral administration of 10 mg of nifedipine. Intrarenal arterial dilatation is evident following the drug

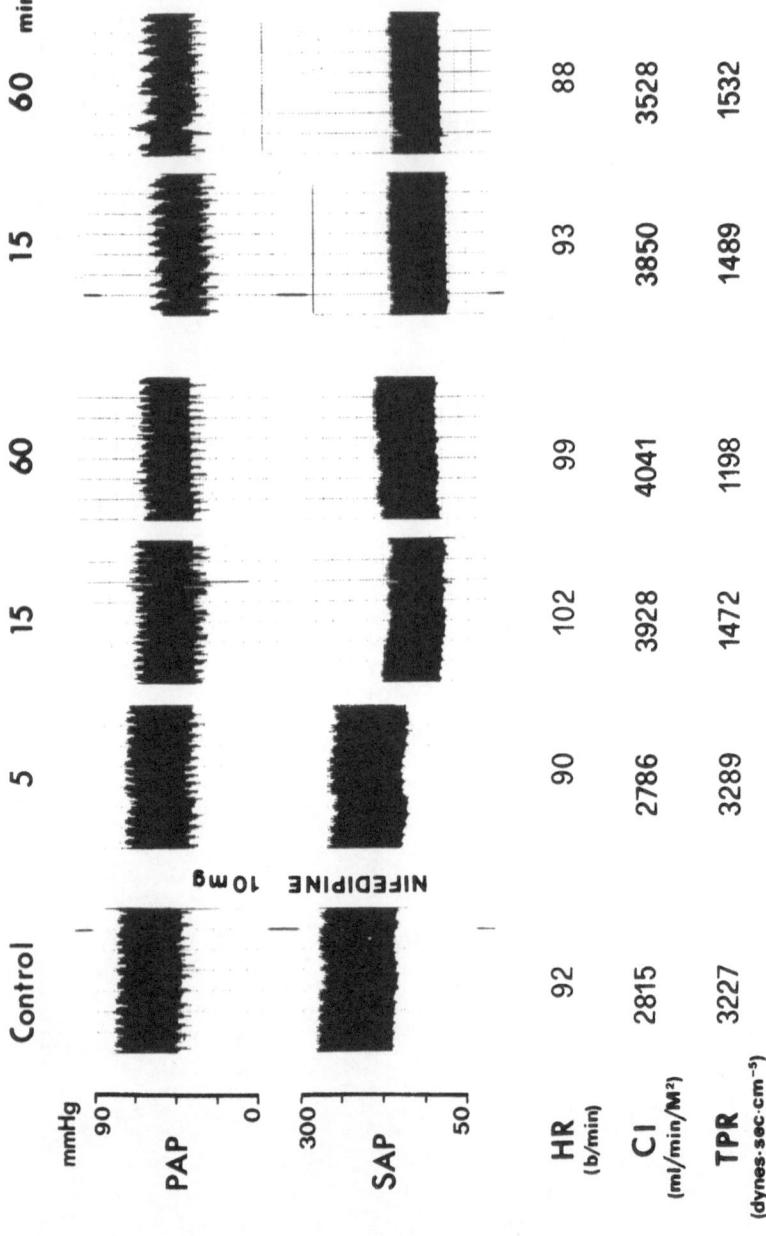

Figure 3 Pulmonary arterial pressure (PAP), systemic arterial pressure (SAP), heart-rate (HR), cardiac index (CI) and total peripheral vascular resistance (TPR) in the control state and at various periods following repeated sublingual administration of nifedipine, in a hypertensive patient with acute left ventricular failure

The drug does not interfere with the sympathetic function. Side-effects, such as short-lasting palpitation, burning sensation in the face, and sporadic premature ventricular contractions, are of infrequent occurrence. In our own experience[39], repeated doses of nifedipine greatly benefited patients with accelerated severe hypertension complicated by encephalopathy or acute left ventricular failure (Figure 3).

Nifedipine may have the same indication in hypertensive emergencies as diazoxide. Advantages of nifedipine are prompt effectiveness by the oral or sublingual route, indication in cases with cardiac ischaemia or insufficiency, and insignificant side-effects.

References

1　Wilson, W. R. and Okun, R. (1963). The acute hemodynamic effects of diazoxide in man. *Circulation*, **28,** 89

2　Hamby, W. M., Jankowski, G. J., Pouget, M., Dunea, G. and Gantt, C. L. (1968). Intravenous use of diazoxide in the treatment of severe hypertension. *Circulation*, **37,** 169

3　Mayler, W. G., McInnes, I., Swann, J. B., Race, D., Carson, V., and Lowe, T. E. (1968). Some effects of the hypotensive drug diazoxide on the cardiovascular system. *Am. Heart J.*, **75,** 223

4　Thirwell, M. P. and Zsoter, T. T. (1972). The effect of diazoxide on the veins. *Am. Heart J.*, **83,** 512

5　Wohl, A. J., Hausler, L. M. and Roth, F. E. (1968). Mechanism of the antihypertensive effect of diazoxide: *in vitro* vascular studies in the hypertensive rat. *J. Pharmacol. Exp. Ther.*, **162,** 109

6　Rubin, A. A., Zitowitz, L. and Hausler, L. (1963). Acute circulatory effects of diazoxide and sodium nitrate. *J. Pharmacol. Exp. Ther.*, **140,** 46

7　Finnerty, F. A. Jr, Kakaviatos, N., Tuckman, J. and Magill, J. (1963). Clinical evaluation of diazoxide. A new treatment for acute hypertension. *Circulation*, **28,** 203

8　Bathia, S. K. and Frohlich, E. D. (1973). Hemodynamic comparison of agents useful in hypertensive emergencies. *Am. Heart J.*, **85,** 367

9　Limbourgh, P., Fiegel, P., Just, H. and Lang, K. F. (1975). Effect of diazoxide on left ventricular performance in hypertension. *Europ. J. Clin. Pharmacol.*, **8,** 387

10　Gifford, R. W. Jr (1974). The management of hypertensive crisis. In W. W. Cabs (ed.). *Critical Care Medicine*, pp. 341–352. (New York: Grune and Stratton)

11　Lockwood, C. H., Nicholis, D. M., Troop, V. L. and Lewis, J. A. (1963). Diazoxide therapy in hypertension. *Am. J. Med. Sci.*, **246,** 312

12　Bateson, M. C. (1976). Postural effect of diazoxide. *Br. Med. J.*, **2,** 698

13　Bartorelli, C., Gargano, N., Leonetti, G. and Zanchetti, A. (1963). Hypotensive and renal effects of diazoxide, a sodium-retaining benzothiazide compound. *Circulation*, **27,** 895

14　Thomson, A. E., Nickerson, M., Gaskell, P. and Grahame, G. R. (1962). Clinical observations on an antihypertensive chlorothiazide devoid of diuretic activity. *Can. Med. Ass. J.*, **87,** 1306

15　Kanada, S. A., Kanada, D. J., Hutchinson, R. A. and Wu, D. (1976). Angina-like syndrome with diazoxide therapy for hypertensive crisis. *Ann. Intern. Med.*, **84,** 696

16 Kumar, G. K., Dastoor, F. C., Robayo, J. R. and Razzaque, M. A. (1976). Side effects of diazoxide. *J. Am. Med. Assoc.*, **235**, 275

17 Paz, M. A., and Sefter, S. (1972). Immunological studies of collagens modified by reaction with hydralazine. *Am. J. Med. Sci.*, **263**, 281

18 Oates, J. A., Gillespie, L., Undenfriend, S. and Sjoerdsma, A. (1960). Decarboxilase inhibition and blood pressure reduction by -methyl-3,4-dihydroxy-DL-phenylalanine. *Science*, **131**, 1890

19 Sannerstedt, R. and Conway, J. (1970). Hemodynamic and vascular responses to antihypertensive treatment with adrenergic blocking agents: a review. *Am. Heart J.*, **79**, 122

20 Bierman, H. D. and Partridge, J. W. (1951). Untoward reactions to tests for epinephrine-secreting tumors (Pheochromocytoma). *N. Engl. J. Med.*, **244**, 582

21 Green, H. D. and Grimsley, W. T. (1953). Effects of regitine (C-7337) in patients, particularly those with peripheral arterial vascular disease. *Circulation*, **7**, 487

22 Taylor, S. H., Sutherland, G. R., McKenzie, G. J., Staunton, H. P. and Donald, K. W. (1965). The circulatory effects of intravenous phentolamine in man. *Circulation*, **31**, 741

23 Cohn, J. N. (1966). Paroxysmal hypertension and hypovolemia. *N. Engl. J. Med.*, **275**, 643

24 Guazzi, M., Fiorentini, C., Polese, A., and Magrini, F. (1973). Hemodynamic factors conditioning the hypotensive response to phentolamine. Limitations of the test in the screening of pheochromocytoma. *Jap. Heart J.*, **14**, 1

25 Guiha, N. H., Cohn, J. N., Mikulic, E., Lima, C. J. and Franciosa, J. A. (1974). Treatment of refractory heart failure with infusion of nitroprusside. *N. Engl. J. Med.*, **291**, 587

26 Miller, R. R., Vismara, L. A., Zelis, R., Amsterdam, E. A. and Mason, D. T. (1975). Clinical use of sodium nitroprusside in chronic ischemic heart disease. *Circulation*, **51**, 328

27 Palmer, R. F. and Lasseter, K. C. (1975). Sodium nitroprusside. *N. Engl. J. Med.*, **292**, 294

28 Shah, P. K. (1977). Ventricular unloading in the management of heart disease: Role of vasodilators. Part 1. *Am. Heart J.*, **93**, 256

29 Freis, E. D. (1969). Hypertensive crisis. *J. Am. Med. Assoc.*, **208**, 338

30 Woods, J. W. and Blythe, W. B. (1967). Management of malignant hypertension complicated by renal insufficiency. *N. Engl. J. Med.*, **277**, 57

31 Woods, J. W., Blythe, W. B. and Huffines, W. D. (1974). Management of malignant hypertension complicated by renal insufficiency. A follow-up study. *N. Engl. J. Med.*, **291**, 10

32 Mutterperl, R. E., Diamond, F. B. and Lowenthal, D. T. (1976). Long-term effects of minoxidil in the treatment of malignant hypertension in chronic renal failure. *J. Clin. Pharmacol.*, **16**, 498

33 Boakes, A. J., Knight, E. J. and Pritchard, B. N. C. (1971). Preliminary studies of the pharmacological effects of (5-1(1-hydroxy-2-[(-1-methyl-3-phenyl propyl amino) ethyl] salicylamide) (AH 5158) in man. *Clin. Sci.*, **40**, 18

34 Farmer, J. B., Kennedy, I., Levy, J. P. and Marshall, R. J. (1972). Pharmacology of AH 5158: A drug which blocks both alpha and beta adreno-receptors. *Br. J. Pharmacol.*, **45**, 660

35 Mehta, J. and Cohn, J. N. (1977). Hemodynamic effects of labetalol, an alpha and beta adrenergic blocking agent, in hypertensive subjects. *Circulation*, **55**, 370

36 Koch, G. (1977). Acute hemodynamic effects of an alpha- and beta-receptor blocking agent (AH 5158) on the systemic and pulmonary circulation at rest and during

exercise in hypertensive patients. *Am. Heart J.*, **93,** 585
37 Agabiti Rosei, E., Brown, J. J., Lever, A. F., Robertson, A. S., Robertson, S. I. S. and Trust, P. M. (1976). Treatment of pheochromocytoma and of clonidine withdrawal hypertension with labetalol. *Br. J. Clin. Pharmacol.*, **3** (4 suppl.), 809
38 Lochner, W., Braasch, W. and Kronenberg, G. (eds.). (1975). *New Therapy of Ischemic Heart Disease* (New York: Springer-Verlag)
39 Guazzi, M., Olivari, M. T., Polese, A., Fiorentini, C., Magrini, F. and Moruzzi, P. (1977). Nifedipine, a new antihypertensive with rapid action. *Clin. Pharmacol. Ther.*, **22,** 528

Toxaemia of Pregnancy

INTRODUCTION: DIAGNOSIS

Hypertension complicates pregnancy in 5–10% of cases. About two-thirds of patients presenting with an elevated blood pressure suffer from a chronic disorder, the aetiology of which is unrelated to pregnancy; one-third develop a disease peculiar to pregnancy which commences during late gestation and subsides following delivery. This disorder is currently called toxaemia of pregnancy, even though no toxin has been discovered in connection with it. The differentiation of chronic hypertension from acute toxaemia is important, since both maternal and fetal prognosis are quite different in the two states. In some cases the differentiation is feasible during pregnancy, but in others precise recognition must await termination of pregnancy. The fact that chronic hypertension can be complicated by an exacerbation during gestation is an additional element of confusion. Recently, the various form of hypertension during pregnancy have been classified by the American College of Obstetricians and Gynecologists[1] as follows:

1 *Mild gestational disorders:*
   (a) gestational or transient hypertension;
   (b) gestational oedema;
   (c) gestational proteinuria
2 *Acute toxaemia:* pre-eclampsia and eclampsia.
3 *Chronic hypertensive disease of whatever cause*
4 *Chronic hypertension with superimposed pre-eclampsia or eclampsia*
5 *Hypertensive disease with insufficient information to allow classification*

For early recognition and proper treatment, the circulatory disorders that may complicate pregnancy, changes in the cardiovascular system associated with normal pregnancy, must be known and the mechanisms for their development understood. This is especially true of cardiologists who are consulted to assist with circulatory problems occurring during pregnancy.

HAEMODYNAMIC CHANGES IN NORMAL PREGNANCY

Exceptional demands are made on the circulation during pregnancy; the heart adapts itself to the raised demands through an increase in output[2]. By the 5th to 6th month of gestation cardiac output is increased by about 8%; by the 7th month it is increased by about 14%, and by term it is increased by about 30–40%. The increase in cardiac output is due, in almost equal proportion, to an increase in heart-rate and stroke volume. The mean blood pressure is unaltered, the diastolic pressure is reduced, peripheral resistance is lowered.

The rise of cardiac output alone is not sufficient to maintain a steady state of the circulation in the presence of the raised capacity of the vascular bed in pregnancy; an increase in circulating blood volume is consequently needed. The total amount of the circulating protein rises proportionally to the increase in the plasma volume, so that the oncotic pressure of the blood remains unchanged[3]; the increase begins during the first 3 months, reaches the maximal value by the 30th week, remains at this level until delivery, and then gradually reverts to normal. The need to raise the volume of the circulating blood leads to an increase in the amount of water in the organism of the pregnant woman. The amounts of solutes rise in parallel with water. The kidney is obviously involved in this positive water and electrolyte balance: during the first 3 months the renal blood flow rises by about 25%, the glomerular filtration rate rises by 50% and remains elevated throughout the pregnancy[4], which results in a higher filtration fraction. The augmented tubular reabsorption of sodium and water is apparently determined by humoral factors, and becomes greater during the last phase of pregnancy. Probably the impeded venous return to the heart from the lower part of the body is a mechanism of potentiation of this effect. The enhanced tendency to a positive salt balance, in association with the increase of hydrostatic pressure in the lower limbs, provides reasonable explanation for the slight oedema of the legs, ankles and feet which develops during the last phase of normal pregnancy in 40% of the cases.

In normal pregnancy, plasma concentration of renin, renin substrate, angiotensin II, and aldosterone are usually increased[5].

GESTATIONAL OR TRANSIENT HYPERTENSION

Transient hypertension is a newly recognized entity in which mild hypertension without proteinuria and oedema develops during pregnancy, but disappears within a few days following delivery. It represents a poorly defined entity which probably includes patients suffering from mild preeclampsia, as well as others who have labile hypertension that becomes manifest only under the stress of pregnancy. In these cases home recording of blood pressure is mandatory to follow its trend, and ordinarily no therapy is needed.

ACUTE TOXAEMIA

Characteristics
Pre-eclampsia and eclampsia are the two forms of acute toxaemia; convulsions or coma in eclampsia, but not in pre-eclampsia, differentiate the two forms. Acute toxaemia is generally recognized by the appearance of hypertension with proteinuria or oedema, or both, after the 20th week of pregnancy. Although this triad is consistent with the diagnosis of toxaemia, it is not diagnostic. In fact, it may be found in pregnant women suffering from various diseases, such as pyelonephritis, glomerulonephritis or hypertensive vascular disease. Pyelonephritis has an elevated frequency in pregnant subjects[6], and an accurate screening for this disease cannot be over-emphasized. The differentiation obviously has important therapeutic and prognostic implications. Fundoscopic examination reveals retinal artery spasm in toxaemia which may provide useful diagnostic information. A role in predicting the development of pregnancy-induced hypertension has recently been attributed to the pressor response to the angiotensin[7] and to the 'roll-over'[8] tests.

Hypertension is said to be present when systolic and diastolic readings are repeatedly higher than 140 and 90 mmHg, respectively. For diagnostic purposes proteinuria is defined as 0.3 grams or more of protein per litre; lesser amounts of proteinuria are relatively common during normal pregnancy. Oedema is less sharply defined; swelling of ankles and feet may be due merely to gravitational causes, while swelling of the hands and periorbital areas can be labelled oedema. Differentiation of mild from severe pre-eclampsia is based on the severity of symptoms and signs, and is not always easy. However, pre-eclampsia need not be severe to progress to eclampsia, and consequently it is safe to institute treatment as soon as diagnosis of pre-eclampsia has been established. A coagulation index based on the platelet count, plasma-factor-VII and serum-fibrinolytic degradation products, seems to be of value in monitoring the progress of the disease[9].

The cause of toxaemia of pregnancy is unknown. Various factors have been indicated. These include changes in the uterus, slow development of intravascular coagulation induced by the release of thromboplastic material into the circulation, renin–angiotensin system[10], and immunological processes[11]. There is no clear evidence, however, that any of these is the primary event in the disease process.

More is known about the pathophysiology of the disease resulting after the exciting factor has had its effect. A generalized capillary disturbance, low filtration fraction, sodium and water retention, vasoconstriction, inadequate amount of the blood proteins and of the circulating blood volume[12] are the major alterations in toxaemia. Their interrelation, as well as their specific role in producing the major features of pre-eclampsia and eclampsia (oedema, proteinuria, hypertension and neurological symptoms), are still conjectural.

TREATMENT

Incipient or mild pre-eclampsia

In this condition, which is signalled by excessive weight gain and slight increase in blood pressure, management at home may be permissible, with more frequent office visits in order to detect any deterioration. Weight gain and slight hypertension may disappear if the patient rests in bed much of the time, limits her sodium intake, and takes a mild sedative, primarily to enforce the bed rest. Prescription of diuretic drugs is a matter of dispute which needs clarification. They should not be prescribed to all pregnant patients with oedema, the amount of which is within the limits described as physiological changes of pregnancy. The administration of diuretics to these patients, whose plasma volume is generally normal, may cause harm to the mother and to the fetus. Only when swelling involves the hands and the periorbital areas, and is associated with some increase in blood pressure, should prescription of diuretics (thiazides) be taken into consideration. The rational basis for their use is that diuretics administered in the early, sodium-retaining phase of pre-eclampsia, should decrease the plasma volume to normal and thus prevent the development of the subsequent vasoconstrictive phase[6]. Views and results, however, are conflicting on this subject.

Severe pre-eclampsia

If the clinical signs are overt and the diagnosis of pre-eclampsia is definitely established, hospitalization is essential.

Termination of pregnancy is the only effective therapeutic modality known for treatment of the woman with pregnancy-induced hypertension. The majority of them develop hypertension late in pregnancy at a time when the fetus is mature, and delivery can be safely effected. There is, however, an appreciable number of women who manifest pre-eclampsia earlier, when the fetus is too immature to survive. In them postponement of delivery would be justified, provided that delay is without significant detrimental consequences to the mother or to the fetus. Favourable results may be achieved by appropriate therapeutic management. Bed rest, sedation, constant clinical monitoring (determination of blood pressure, body weight, urine protein, creatinine clearance, serial sonography) and continued medical correction of the pathological changes of the disease (hypertension, sodium retention, oliguria, hypovolaemia) represent the main aspects of management. These procedures are most effectively carried out in a high-risk pregnancy unit[13].

Blood pressure must be normalized, and specific drug therapy instituted when elevated levels do not subside with bed rest alone. Provided that a normovolaemic state exists or has been restored, thiazides and related drugs are the mainstay of treatment. Reserpine, hydralazine, or methyldopa may be added when thiazides are not completely effective. For most patients reserpine (0.25 mg) is the drug of choice; if the response is poor, methyldopa can be substituted. When reserpine or methyldopa induce over-sedation, the combination of thiazide with hydralazine may be preferable. A successful use of oral diazoxide in the treatment of severe toxaemia has been reported[14]. Long-term prescription of this compound in pregnancy, however, has been criticized[15].

Eclampsia
Though hypertension is not invariably associated with eclampsia, the most common cause of death is cerebral haemorrhage complicating the acute hypertensive episode. In eclampsia the therapeutic aims are: preventing or controlling convulsions without causing harm to the fetus; reducing the diastolic pressure continuously to under 90 mmHg; maintaining the urinary output above 1500 ml/24 h. Sedative and tranquillizing compounds have poor or no effect on hypertension, unless they are administered in anaesthetic doses; combination of specific antihypertensive preparations is a much more rational approach.

When antihypertensive treatment for acute eclampsia is being instituted, two concepts should be kept in mind: (1) eclampsia is characterized by sodium retention, and decrease in blood volume, renal blood flow and urinary output; (2) acute reduction of arterial pressure is associated with transient reduction of glomerular filtration rate, renal blood flow and urinary output, resulting in further sodium retention. Hydralazine, nitroprusside or diazoxide (given for short periods by intermittent intravenous injections) are the drugs of choice for treating hypertensive emergencies of eclampsia. Their association with diuretics (furosemide) is essential to increase the urinary output and reduce sodium retention. Diuretics are effective and, indeed, should be used only when a normovolaemic state exists; if the patient presents with hypovolaemia, a normal circulatory volume should be restored. Central venous pressure monitoring may provide an important aid for the achievement of a normovolaemic state[16].

After the eclamptic woman has been stabilized by these measures, delivery should be accomplished in 6–12 h. This interval is utilized to ensure that the patient will have achieved optimal condition for terminating pregnancy by Caesarian section.

CHRONIC HYPERTENSIVE DISEASE IN PREGNANCY

Chronic hypertensive disease in pregnancy is usually due to essential hypertension, to chronic pyelonephritis or, less often, to chronic glomerulonephritis. Many other diseases are rare causes of hypertension: collagen disease, diabetic nephropathy or phaeochromocytoma. When pregnancy occurs in a patient with chronic hypertension, careful evaluation and monitoring are necessary; the indications for hypotensive treatment, and the therapeutic regimen, are the same as though the patient were not pregnant. The outcome depends primarily on the extent of the original organ damage, notably of the kidney, and on the superposition of acute toxaemia in certain patients. While many subjects with chronic hypertension progress through pregnancy without difficulty, some will require therapeutic abortion or even renal dialysis[17] in order to survive. Fetal or neonatal death is a common occurrence in these patients.

References

1 Hughes, E. C. (1972). *Obstetric–Gynecologic Terminology* (Philadelphia: Davies)

2 Hamilton, B. E. (1954). Cardiovascular problems in pregnancy. *Circulation*, **9**, 922

3 Freis, E. D. and Kenny, J. F. (1948). Plasma volume, total circulatory protein and 'available fluid' abnormalities in preeclampsia. *J. Clin. Invest.*, **27**, 283

4 Bucht, H. (1951). Studies on renal function in man with special reference to glomerular filtration and renal plasma flow in pregnancy. *Scand. J. Clin. Lab. Invest.*, **3** (Suppl.), 1

5 Weir, R. J., Paintin, D. B. and Robertson J. I. S. (1970). Renin, angiotensin, aldosterone relationship in normal pregnancy. *Proc. R. Soc. Med.*, **63**, 1101

6 Finnerty, F. A. (1964). Clinical hemodynamics and pharmacodynamics of toxemia. *Circulation*, **29** and **30** (Suppl. 2), 63

7 Gant, N. F., Daley, G. L., Chand, S., Whalley, P. J. and MacDonald, P. C. (1973). A study of angiotensin II pressor response throughout primigravid pregnancy. *J. Clin. Invest.*, **52**, 2682

8 Gusdon, J. P. Jr, Anderson, S. G. and May W. J. (1977). A clinical evaluation of the 'roll-over test' for pregnancy-induced hypertension. *Am. J. Obstet. Gynecol.*, **127**, 1

9 Howie, P. W., Begg, C. B., Purdie, D. W. and Prentice, C. R. M. (1976). Use of coagulation tests to predict the clinical progress of pre-eclampsia. *Lancet*, **2**, 323

10 Hypertension in pregnancy. (1975). *Lancet*, **2**, 487

11 Immunological factors in pre-eclampsia. (1976). *Br. Med. J.*, **2**, 604

12 Soffronoff, E. C., Kauffmann, B. M. and Connaughton, J. F. (1977). Intravascular volume determinations and fetal outcome in hypertensive diseases of pregnancy. *Am. J. Obstet. Gynecol.*, **127**, 4

13 Hauth, J. C., Cunningham, F.G. and Whalley, P. J. (1976). Management of pregnancy-induced hypertension in the nullipara. *Obstet. Gynecol.*, **48**, 253

14 Pohl, J. E. F., Thurston, H., Davies, D. and Morgan, M. Y. (1972). Successful use of oral diazoxide in the treatment of severe toxemia of pregnancy. *Br. Med. J.*, **1**, 568

15 Perkins, R. P. (1976). Diazoxide in treatment of severe pre-eclampsia and hypertensive encephalopathy. *Am. J. Obstet. Gynecol.*, **126**, 296

16 McLean, A. B., Doig, J. R., and Aickin, D. R. (1976). Management of eclampsia. *Br. Med. J.*, **2**, 368

17 Schreiner, G. E. (1976). Dialysis and pregnancy. *J. Am. Med. Assoc.*, **236**, 1725

Renal Hypertension

INTRODUCTION

High blood pressure is a cardinal manifestation of renal disease. As hypertension may accompany, with varying frequency, almost any disease of the kidney, there is little to be gained from attempting to make an exhaustive list of renal disorders which may cause hypertension. An arrangement in groups, however, may facilitate the analysis of the therapeutic aspects of various forms of renal hypertension. The following classification is proposed:

1 *Hypertension due to parenchymal renal disease* (glomerulonephritis, pyelonephritis and, less commonly, polycystic disease, diabetic nephropathy, analgesic nephropathy, amyloidosis and collagen disease);

2 *Hypertension due to urologic disease* (obstructive uropathy deriving from prostatic hypertrophy, ureteral stones, bladder tumours, retroperitoneal fibrosis);

3 *Hypertension of end-stage renal disease;*

4 *Reno-vascular hypertension* (atherosclerotic renal artery stenosis, fibromuscular dysplasia, renal artery compression by haemato-

ma, cysts, tumours, retroperitoneal fibrosis and arterovenous
fistulas of the renal artery).

Management of hypertension in acute and chronic renal disease
requires knowledge of the haemodynamics in the various situations,
understanding of the importance of salt and water balance, vaso-
pressor function of the diseased kidney, information on the effects
of pharmacological agents on haemodynamics as well as on renal
function. Renal hypertension can, like essential hypertension, be
treated with modern hypotensive drugs; the difference between the
two diseases, however, must be borne in mind. In essential hypertension, at least in the initial stage, the kidneys are morphologically
intact and the renal blood flow does not fall with the pressure drop,
but may actually increase. In hypertension of renal origin, in which
the size of the vascular bed and its capability of prompt adjustment to
blood pressure changes are reduced, the possibility of deterioration of
renal blood flow must obviously be taken into account.

HAEMODYNAMIC AND RENAL EFFECTS OF ANTIHYPERTENSIVE AGENTS

Diuretics

Thiazides reduce systolic and diastolic pressures in proportional
amounts, induce little or no postural hypotension and produce no
major changes in regional blood flows. According to the current in-
terpretation the short-term antihypertensive effect of thiazides is due
primarily to volume depletion, while the long-term effect is ascribed
to a direct relaxant action on arteriolar smooth muscle. Recent haemodynamic findings of Shah and co-workers[1] suggest a unitary
rather than a dual theory of the mode of action of the thiazides.
Reduction of extracellular fluid volume produces initially a fall in
cardiac output associated with an increased total vascular resistance.
However, with continued treatment and maintained reduction in
cardiac output and total blood flow, autoregulation occurs gradually
over a period of weeks leading to a decline in peripheral vascular
resistance; the resulting fall in after-load permits a rise in cardiac
output towards normal. The sequence of the haemodynamic
changes during the early and late phases of continuous treatment
with thiazides can be explained by a single effect which is a sustained reduction in extracellular fluid volume; no direct vasodilator
action needs to be postulated.

The reduction in glomerular filtration rate induced by thiazides may be of clinical importance, particularly in patients with diminished renal reserve[2]. Ethacrynic acid, furosemide and bumetanide form the group of the so-called high ceiling or loop diuretics. These drugs share in common prompt onset of action, inhibition of sodium and chloride transport in the ascending limb of the loop of Henle. Depending on the dose and speed of administration, an increase in renal blood flow, as well as its redistribution within the kidney, may occur: there is generally an increase of blood flow in the cortex, accompanied by a decrease in the outer medulla[3]. Potency and ability to maintain glomerular filtration rate make their use suitable in patients with reduced renal function[4,5]. These agents, like the thiazide diuretics, stimulate renin release from the kidney.

Vasodilators
Hydralazine is the drug of this group which is used more extensively in the treatment of hypertension; its haemodynamic and renal effects have been described in the section on Hypertensive Crisis. A number of other compounds, such as minoxidil and guancydine, distant congeners of hydralazine, appear to have very similar haemodynamic effects and exert considerable antihypertensive activity in man. Minoxidil, in association with furosemide and beta-blockers, was effective in achieving rapid and persistent control of blood pressure in a large number of patients with hypertension associated with chronic renal insufficiency[6]. Nephrectomy could be avoided in cases with end-stage renal disease and refractory hypertension when minoxidil was used to reduce blood pressure[7,8]. Prazosin is another vasodilator which decreases blood pressure and peripheral vascular resistance, with small effect on cardiac output[9] and mild increase in glomerular filtration rate.

Drugs interfering with adrenergic activity
The circulatory effects of reserpine, methyldopa and ganglion-blocking agents have been discussed under Hypertensive Crisis. Guanethidine may be considered representative of drugs that depress the function of post-ganglionic adrenergic fibres. Overall responses after guanethidine administration are resultant of decreased release of adrenergic mediator from sympathetic nerve endings and increased sensitivity of effector cell to the mediator. Intravenous injection of guanethidine results in catecholamine release and a rise of blood pressure. The drug, therefore, should only be administered orally. Its duration of action is very long, so that only a once-daily dosage is indicated. Renal blood flow and glomerular filtration rate

decrease considerably after acute or chronic administration of this compound[10]. Its therapeutic use is somewhat limited because of the prominent orthostatic hypotension.

Reduced sympathetic outflow, due to an action on the central nervous system, is the principal mechanism of the antihypertensive response to clonidine. Acute intravenous administration induces hypotension, bradycardia and cardiac output reduction. Pressure reduction is potentiated by tilting, and is due to a decrease in vascular resistance. Glomerular filtration rate is usually diminished, renal vascular resistance is reduced, renal blood flow is not decreased, sodium excretion is considerably diminished. Following chronic administration blood pressure is usually reduced less than after a single dose, relative bradycardia persists, cardiac output is maintained, plasma renin activity is reduced. Tolerance to the hypotensive effect of clonidine appears less frequent when a diuretic is added.

Beta-adrenergic blockers
Treatment of arterial hypertension with beta-adrenergic blocking agents has become increasingly popular during the last few years. Propranolol, and most of the other beta-adrenergic blockers that are clinically available, could be reported as 'first-generation beta-blockers'. They block both beta-$_1$ receptors, e.g. in the myocardium, and beta-$_2$ receptors, e.g. in the bronchi and peripheral blood vessels. More recently drugs have been developed, such as practolol, metoprolol and atenolol, indicated as 'second-generation beta-blockers' which are characterized by specific beta-$_1$ receptors blockade. Although experience with these newer agents appears promising, further experience is needed before one can state that these compounds are as safe and effective as the 'first-generation beta-blockers'.

The mechanism of their antihypertensive action is still unsettled. Propranolol was initially reported as being effective mainly through a chronic reduction of cardiac output; later it has been shown that a gradual readjustment of vascular resistance towards the initial level or lower takes place during chronic treatment[11]. Changes in blood volume do not seem to be related to this effect. A reduction of the adrenergic outflow due to a depressive effect at the level of the central nervous system has been postulated from findings in animals, but so far it has not been proved in man[12]. That beta-blockers reduce renin release and plasma renin activity has been demonstrated in several studies[13]. Although this may not be the exclusive mechanism of the antihypertensive effect of beta-blockers they are particularly effective in hypertension associated with high levels of renin secretion.

Propranolol has been indicated as the drug of choice in patients with renal hypertension and high plasma renin activity, and its combination with a vasodilator has been recommended as an alternative to nephrectomy in renal hypertension[14]. As with many other antihypertensive agents there may be a temporary reduction of renal blood flow and glomerular filtration rate[15].

TREATMENT OF THE HYPERTENSION

Acute glomerulonephritis

Many clinicians believe that control of blood pressure is important in the management of glomerulonephritis. This is a clinical impression which mostly originates from the favourable effects of treatment in essential hypertension. However, data on the effect of hypertension on survival of patients with glomerulonephritis are quite scanty. A retrospective survey carried out by Sarre *et al.*[16] indicates that those with elevated blood pressure fare worse than those who are normotensive.

Both the oedema and the hypertension in patients with acute glomerulonephritis benefit from restriction of salt intake. If the blood pressure remains elevated and oedema persists, the use of diuretics is indicated. Thiazide derivatives may be used in patients with glomerular filtration rate above 60 ml/min; if the glomerular filtration rate is below this value and azotaemia is present, furosemide or ethacrynic acid should be preferred. Treatment with furosemide may be initiated with a dose of 40 mg three times daily; a progressive increase up to 200 mg three times daily may be necessary in cases of severely impaired renal function. Clonidine, beginning at 0·1 mg twice daily, or methyldopa, at 250 mg twice daily and both titrated upward as needed, should be added if blood pressure is not controlled by the diuretic alone. If the blood pressure reduction is not satisfactory, hydralazine should be added at the dose of 25 mg from two to three times per day and increased if needed to 50 mg three times daily. The three-drug combination achieves satisfactory control of blood pressure in the great majority of cases. A further advantage from this association of drugs is that methyldopa and clonidine moderate the tachycardia elicited by hydralazine. The treatment of hypertensive crisis which may occur in acute glomerulonephritis has been discussed elsewhere.

Unilateral parenchymal renal disease

Little information is available on the cure rate from nephrectomy in the hypertension associated with unilateral renal parenchymal disease. However, reviews of a large number of hypertensive patients with unilateral renal disease who underwent nephrectomy have shown that remission of hypertension after a year was achieved in only a disappointingly low 26%[17] to 37%[18]. Included in these series were patients with renal artery lesions, so that the cure rate in parenchymal disease, *per se*, may be even lower. Recent findings[19] suggest that nephrectomy is only indicated when there is: (1) increased renin secretion; (2) well-defined total contralateral suppression of renin secretion; and (3) abnormally elevated renin-vein to arterial relationship from the involved kidney, indicating flow reduction. In addition, nephrectomy may be indicated in the setting of the totally non-functioning kidney, where there may be a hope for reduction of some renin-secreting potential, without losing any sodium-excretion capacity. In most patients, however, both kidneys will be contributing significantly to the overall renal function. When these criteria are not fulfilled, specific pharmacological treatment, directed at both the vasoconstrictor component by renin secretion inhibitors, such as beta-adrenergic blocking agents, and the volume component by diuretic therapy, takes precedence over a surgical approach.

Chronic renal failure
This group includes patients with impairment of renal function of a moderate to severe degree, but who have not yet reached end-stage renal insufficiency. There are two distinct types of patients: those with chronic renal failure secondary to renal parenchymal disease, such as glomerulonephritis or pyelonephritis, and those characterized by having essential hypertension associated with nephroangiosclerosis. Regardless of the aetiology of the renal lesions, persistent hypertension will contribute significantly to the deterioration of renal blood flow and to the progression of the renal failure by enhancing renal arterial and arteriolar sclerosis. To arrest this process, control of the elevated blood pressure is required.

The use of low-salt diets to control hypertension must be approached cautiously, since some patients with kidney disease (notably when damage of the medulla is predominant) may waste salt. Excessive reduction of salt intake in such patients will result in volume depletion, renal hypoperfusion, and further reduction of glomerular filtration rate. The thiazide diuretics are not indicated in this type of patient because they reduce glomerular filtration rate and also because they are ineffective at low rates of glomerular filtration.

If the patient is not a salt-loser but has advanced renal failure, and if diuretic is indicated, it is usually necessary to use furosemide or ethacrynic acid. The dose of furosemide depends on both the blood pressure level and the degree of reduction of glomerular filtration rate. Patients with glomerular filtration rates reduced to below 30 ml/min may require doses up to 200 mg one to three times a day, or even higher.

When diuretics alone are ineffective, methyldopa or clonidine should be added. Both drugs require dosage titration; both preserve to a certain extent renal blood flow and glomerular filtration rate. Methyldopa is initiated in a dose of 250 mg twice daily and can be progressively increased to 2 g/day. For clonidine the starting dose is 0·1 mg twice daily, which may be progressively increased up to 1 mg twice daily. If hypertension persists hydralazine should be added in a dose of 10–25 mg four times daily; it may be increased to a total dose of 300 mg per day. Propranolol is also effective in the treatment of renal hypertension, and may be used in conjunction with vasodilators such as prazosin[20] and hydralazine[21]. Interference with sexual function, occurrence of orthostatic hypotension, and failure to suppress recumbent blood pressure adequately discourage the use of guanethidine.

End-stage renal disease
Numerous studies document the effectiveness of bilateral nephrectomy to control severe hypertension in selected cases with end-stage renal disease[22,23]. Bilateral nephrectomy has even been advocated in patients with severe hypertension who have not progressed to end-stage renal disease[24]. The recommendation for bilateral nephrectomy to prevent the well-known complications of severe hypertension must be analysed with the utmost care, and the possible benefits must be balanced against the hazards of anaesthesia and surgery in critically-ill subjects and of long-term haemodialysis or renal transplantation.

Several considerations argue against bilateral nephrectomy as an emergency procedure. The observation that some of the patients with azotaemic malignant hypertension may regain a degree of renal function through an adequate trial of medical and dialytic therapy, suggests that some patients would be nephrectomized unnecessarily if renal excision was carried out as an emergency procedure. In addition, the position that immediate nephrectomy will prevent the damages of the elevated pressure is untenable, since the introduction of potent antihypertensive compounds both for acute (diazoxide, trimethaphan, nitroprusside) and long-term (clonidine, minoxidil, propranolol) control of blood pressure. Recent reports have been extremely encouraging in this regard[7–9,20,25]. At the present time, therefore, there is no justification for an emergency bilateral nephrectomy.

When hypertension is moderate, the first step is use of haemodialysis in association with restriction of salt and water intake. If the blood pressure is not controlled, clonidine, methyldopa or hydralazine can be added subsequently, according to the method indicated in the preceding section. Propranolol associated with vasodilators (hydralazine or minoxidil) is an alternative therapeutic regimen.

An adequate trial of medical and dialytic therapy should involve a period of 6–8 months; if a satisfactory control of blood pressure is not achieved, bilateral nephrectomy may then be considered. Earlier nephrectomy is indicated in cases with hypertension in the malignant phase which does not respond promptly to antihypertensive drug treatment, or in patients who cannot tolerate antihypertensive drugs. It is well documented that subjects with hypertensive terminal renal failure, especially those with hyperreninaemia, can be expected to have a general clinical amelioration (reappearance of appetite, sense of well-being, weight gain), and improvement in the control of hypertension after bilateral nephrectomy. If antihypertensive treatment is still required, the principles of administration and selection of drugs are the same as before nephrectomy. The fact that in the anephric state blood pressure becomes extremely sensitive to salt and water balance must be taken into account.

Renovascular hypertension
Renovascular hypertension is surgically correctable. Intense screening for renovascular hypertension deserves some comments. Conventional radiological techniques (intravenous urogram and renogram) when performed routinely in hypertensive subjects reveal a primary renal abnormality in only a minority of cases, and only a fraction of these have a surgically correctable form, the incidence of which has been reported to vary from 1%[26] to 3%[27] of the total hypertensive population.

In assessing the value of intense screening for renovascular hypertension it is also necessary to evaluate the outcome of surgery. If patients are better off with medical treatment, the search for a renal cause is of only academic interest. A recent survey of the published data surprisingly suggests that more patients survived as a result of medical treatment of renovascular hypertension than those who had surgical correction, although there was a slightly greater incidence of non-fatal vascular accidents in the former group[28]. These arguments indicate that the real importance of surgical correctable renal hypertension must be reconsidered. In addition, the economic implications of subjecting every patient with elevated blood pressure to intravenous urography and renography are staggering[29], and strongly suggest the need for less expensive and time-consuming screening investigations.

If the unproved assumption is admitted that elevated blood pressure in surgically correctable hypertension is maintained by the renin–angiotensin system, alternative procedures might be that of the infusion of angiotensin antagonists[30], or converting enzyme inhibitors[31], or that of the measurement of plasma renin activity or concentration[32]. Even if angiotensin antagonists are generally available, there are some reservations about their routine use: in some circumstances they can have distinct vasodepressor action[33,34].

The use of plasma renin measurements is not new, and has met with differing degrees of success. Part of the past discordances and disappointments may find explanation in: inadequate methodology of renin determination; poor control of the variables that influence renin determinations; use of the method to assess surgical curability rather than to filter off patients who require further radiological and biochemical studies; comparison of a given plasma-renin value with a range derived from normal individuals rather than from patients with essential hypertension.

The variables which influence renin determinations are manifold, and it is critically important that these be controlled if renin determinations are to provide clinically useful information. Sodium depletion brought about by dietary restriction, or diuretic drugs, sharply stimulate renin release. Both posture and physical activity stimulate secretion of renin, but posture is more important. Their effects are dissipated after 60–90 min in the supine position. An important influence of the sympathetic nervous system is also recognized[13], which is difficult to assess clinically but may be affected by medications. Compounds which acutely stimulate renin release include all the diuretics and the vasodilating drugs. Inhibitors of renin release include propranolol, methyldopa, reserpine, ganglion-blocking agents and clonidine. Oral contraceptives raise plasma-renin activity by stimulating increased production of substrate. To avoid drug influences at least 7 days should elapse between stopping medication and renin studies, and 60 days in the case of oral contraceptives.

However, adequacy in the methodology of renin determination

and proper control of the variables that may interfere with renin secretion represent obvious difficulties which still limit the use of this method for routine screening in the general practice of medicine.

Rapid-sequence intravenous urogram, renal arteriograms, renal vein renin determinations and, possibly, angiotensin antagonist tests are the subsequent steps for identification of lesions in the renal artery that can cause renovascular hypertension, and for prediction of surgical curability. Major urographic features are disparity in renal length, caliceal appearance time, and concentration on late films. Patients most favourable for surgical cure should have the following: unilateral main renal artery lesion; peripheral plasma-renin activity inappropriately high relative to sodium excretion on constant sodium intake; high renal vein renin release on the involved side (ratio greater than $1 \cdot 5$); suppressed renin release from the opposite kidney (V–A + 0); prompt and significant reduction in blood pressure (more than 35 mm systolic and 25 mm diastolic) with intravenous angiotensin or converting enzyme inhibitors during sodium restriction. Although wide experience and prolonged follow-up are still lacking, experience accumulated in the past few years suggests that patients meeting all, or nearly all, of these criteria, have a high likelihood of surgical cure[36]. An appropriate surgical repair in patients with definite ischaemia and without significant atherosclerotic disease and complications can produce worthwhile results.

After determination of significant renal ischaemia, surgery should be performed only when the patient is not more than 55 years of age, the function of the uninvolved kidney is at least 50% of normal, the patient has no significant peripheral vascular disease and has not had myocardial infarction or cerebral vascular accident previously, and frank diabetes is absent. Patients who do not meet these criteria should be treated medically, even if they present significant ischaemia of the involved kidney. When medical therapy is inadequate for control, or compliance to treatment is poor, or the disease is progressing, surgery could be justified in such patients, although amelioration rather than cure should be expected.

References

1 Shah, S., Khatri, I. and Freis, E. D. (1978). Mechanism of antihypertensive effect of thiazide diuretics. *Am. Heart J.*, **95**, 611

2 Gifford, R. W. (1959). Chlorthiazide in the treatment of hypertension. *Postgrad. Med. J.*, **25**, 559

3 Hook, J. B., Blatt, A. H., Brody, M. J. and Williamsons, H. E. (1966). Effects of several saluretic-diuretic agents on renal hemodynamics. *J. Pharmacol. Exp. Ther.*, **154**, 667

4 Berman, L. B. and Ebrahimi, A. (1965). Experiences with furosemide in renal disease. *Proc. Soc. Exp. Biol. Med.*, **118**, 333

5 Muth, R. G. (1966). Diuretic response to furosemide in the presence of renal insufficiency. *J. Am. Med. Assoc.*, **195**, 1066

6 Mutterperl, R. E., Frayda, D. O., Diamond, R. N. and Lowenthal, D. T. (1976). Long-term effects of minoxidil in the treatment of malignant hypertension in chronic renal failure. *J. Clin. Pharmacol.*, **16**, 498

7 Pettinger, W. A. and Mitchell, H. C. (1973). Minoxidil — an alternative to nephrectomy for refractory hypertension. *N. Engl. J. Med.*, **289**, 167

8 Lima, C. J. and Freis, E. D. (1973). Minoxidil in severe hypertension with renal failure. *Am. J. Cardiol.*, **31**, 355

9 Fernandes, M., Smith, I. S., Wender, A., Kim, K. E., Gould, A. B., Busby, P., Swartz, C., and Onesti, G. (1975). Prazosin in the treatment of hypertension. *Clin. Sci. Mol. Med.*, **48**, 181s

10 Richardson, D. W., Myso, E. M., Magee, J. H. and Cavell, G. C. (1960). Circulatory effects of guanethidine. Clinical, renal and cardiac responses with a novel antihypertensive drug. *Circulation*, **22**, 184

11 Tarazi, R. C. and Dustan, H. C. (1972). Beta-adrenergic blockade in hypertension: practical and theoretical implications of long-term hemodynamic variations. *Am. J. Cardiol.*, **29**, 633

12 Guazzi, M., Fiorentini, C., Polese, A., Olivari, M. T. and Magrini, F. (1976). Antihypertensive action of propranolol in man: lack of evidence for a neural depressive effect. *Clin. Pharmacol. Ther.*, **20**, 304

13 Zanchetti, A., Stella, A., Leonetti, G., Morganti, A. and Terzoli, L. (1976). Control of renin release: a review of experimental evidence and clinical implications. *Am. J. Cardiol.*, **37**, 675

14 New vasodilator drugs for hypertension (1973). *Br. Med. J.*, **4**, 185

15 Ibsen, H. and Sederberg-Olsen, P. (1973). Changes in glomerular filtration rate during long-term treatment with propranolol in patients with arterial hypertension *Clin. Sci.*, **44**, 129

16 Sarre, H., Kluthe, R., Jerdinsky, H. J., Baum, P., Buchborne, E., Durr, F., Edel, H., Fritz, K. W., Heidland, A., Heintz, R., Jutzler, G. A., Kortze, P., Kreche, H. J., Lange, W., Nieth, H., Oberwittler, J., Oechslen, D., Portwich, P., Schirmeister, J., Schutterle, G., Sieberth, H. G. and Wetzeis, E. (1971). Nephrotisches syndrom des erwachsenenalters. *Dtsch. Med. Wochenschr.*, **96**, 225

17 Smith, H. W. (1956). Unilateral nephrectomy in hypertensive disease. *J. Urol.*, **76**, 685

18 Kincaid-Smith, P. (1961). Renal ischemia and hypertension: a review of results of surgery. *Australas. Ann. Med.*, **10**, 166

19 Vaughan, D. E. Jr, Buhler, F. R., Laragh, J. H., Sealey, J. E., Gavras, H. and Baer, L. (1975). Hypertension and unilateral parenchymal renal disease. Evidence for abnormal vasoconstriction–volume interaction. *J. Am. Med. Assoc.*, **233**, 1177

20 Curtis, J. R. and Bateman, F. J. A. (1975). Use of prazosin in management of hypertension in patients with chronic renal failure and in renal transplant recipients. *Br. Med. J.*, **4**, 432

21 Kincaid-Smith, P. (1974). Beta-adrenergic blocking agents in renal failure. *Br. Med. J.*, **3**, 520

22 Mahony, J. F., Storey, G. B., Gibson, G. R., Stokes, G. S., Sheil, A. G. R. and Stewart, J. H. (1972). Bilateral nephrectomy for malignant hypertension.

Lancet, **1,** 1036

23 Kim, K. E., Onesti, G., Schwartz, A. B., Chinitz, J. L. and Swartz, C. (1972) Hemodynamics of hypertension in chronic end-stage renal disease. *Circulation,* **46,** 456

24 Lazarus, J. M.,   Hampers, C. L.,   Bennett, A. H.,   Vandam, L. D.   and Merrill, J. P. (1972). Urgent bilateral nephrectomy for severe hypertension. *Ann. Intern. Med.,* **76,** 733

25 Buhler, F. R.,   Laragh, J. H.,   Bauer, L.,   Vaughan, E. D. Jr,   and Brunner, H. R. (1972). Propranolol inhibition of renin secretion: a specific approach to diagnosis and treatment of renin-dependent hypertensive disease. *N. Engl. J. Med.,* **287,** 1209

26 Bech, K. and Hilten, T. (1975). The frequency of secondary hypertension. *Acta Med. Scand.,* **197,** 65

27 Bailey, S. M., Evans, D. W. and Fleming, H. A. (1975). Intravenous urography in investigation of hypertension. *Lancet,* **2,** 57

28 McNeil, B. J. and Adelstein, S. J. (1975). The value of case finding in hypertensive renovascular disease. *N. Engl. J. Med.,* **293,** 221

29 McNeil, B. J., Varady, P. D., Burrows, B. A. and Adelstein, S. J. (1975). Cost-effectiveness calculations in the diagnosis and treatment of hypertensive renovascular disease. *N. Engl. J. Med.,* **293,** 216

30 Streeten, D. H. P., Anderson, G. H., Freiberg, J. M. and Dalakos, T. G. (1975). Use of angiotensin II antagonist (saralasin) in the recognition of 'angiotensinogenic' hypertension. *N. Engl. J. Med.,* **292,** 657

31 Case, D. B., Wallace, J. M., Keim, H. J., Weber, M. A., Drayer, J. I., White, R. P. and Laragh, J. H. (1976). Estimating renin participation in hypertension: superiority of converting enzyme inhibitor over saralasin. *Am. J. Med.,* **61,** 790

32 Page, L. B. (1976). Clinical value of plasma renin determination in renovascular and primary hypertension. *Am. Heart J.,* **91,** 665

33 Pettinger, W. A. and Keeton, K. (1975). Hypotension during angiotensin blockade with saralasin. *Lancet,* **1,** 1387

34 Beckerhoff, R., Furrer, J., Vetter, W., Nussberger, J. and Siegenthaler, W. (1976). Hypotension during angiotensin blockade with saralasin. *Br. Med. J.,* **2,** 349

35 Swales, J. D. (1976). The hunt for renal hypertension. *Lancet,* **1,** 577

36 Laragh, J. H., Sealey, J. E., Buhler, R. F., Vaughn, E.D., Brunner, H. R., Gravas, H. and Baer, L. (1975). The renin axis and vasoconstrictor volume analysis for understanding and treating renovascular hypertension. *Am. J. Med.,* **58,** 4

7

The compliance problem in hypertension

F. A. Finnerty Jr.

INTRODUCTION

Diagnosing hypertension is quite easy, e.g., recording the arterial pressure takes less than a minute; and treating most patients, at least those with mild disease, is usually quite simple, e.g., taking a pill a day. The problem is how to keep asymptomatic patients under medical care and on medication. The advances in therapy are not going to be realized; strokes, congestive heart failure, heart attacks, and renal failure are not going to be prevented – unless the patient takes his medication and stays under medical care.

It must be emphasized at the beginning that the problem of non-compliance in hypertension is relatively new. The prevalence of high blood pressure was not determined until the 1960s; the rationale for lowering blood pressure was not established until the Veterans Administration Cooperative Studies in 1967 and 1970; and the problem of non-compliance has only been generally recognized since 1972.

CAUSES OF NON-COMPLIANCE

There are many factors responsible for poor compliance:

1 Long waiting-times in overcrowded areas (particularly in clinics), not only waiting for the physician but also standing in line at the pharmacy.
2 Poor follow-up.
3 Complicated treatment schedules.
4 Side-effects.
5 A poor or non-existent doctor–patient relationship.

151

Study of a large out-patient clinic

In order to gain an insight into the tremendous problem of patient non-compliance, a sociologist and I recently conducted a survey among patients who dropped out from hypertension clinics in an inner city[1]. We rapidly learned that patients dropped out not because they were un-educated or did not care about their health, and not because they could not afford the medication.

Rather, they abandoned the clinic because they were treated like cattle, herded from one room to another, left waiting for hours, then ex-amined by a different doctor on each visit, leaving no opportunity to de-velop any kind of a relationship. Their major complaints centred around two points:

(a) The many wasted hours they spent at the clinic.
(b) The lack of a personal relationship.

The average waiting time for the doctor was 2·5 h, and the average waiting time for drugs at the pharmacy was another 1·8 h. Since most of the patients used public transportation, travel time was considered as one more frustrating element of the problem.

In contrast to the long waiting-time before and after the examination, the average time actually spent with the physician was only 7·5 min. This was obviously not enough time for the patient to have questions an-swered, to learn about his disease, or to begin to establish a good doctor–patient relationship. The fact that the patient was examined by a different physician on each visit decreased the chances of the patient developing any type of a personal relationship. Our group reorganized the hypertension clinic using the patient's complaints as guidelines. There were three major objectives:

1 To develop a meaningful appointment system.
2 To develop a real personal relationship with the patient.
3 To provide convenient service for the patient.

Instead of operating a Monday morning clinic with all the patients coming in at 7.30 a.m. and the physicians arriving at 9.30 or 10 a.m., the patient was given a definite appointment at 8.30 or 9.15 a.m. The day before the scheduled appointment the patient would be notified. Simi-larly if the patient did not keep his appointment he was contacted im-mediately and scheduled for another one.

Most important was the assignment of every patient to his or her own paramedic whom he would see on every visit. The paramedics frequently came from the same neighbourhood as the patient, and therefore knew who to call 'Honey' or who to call Mr Jones'. Each of the paramedics received on-the-job training and was chosen not so much because of her prior experience or education but because of her friendly and sympathetic personality and ability to identify with the patients.

The wait at the pharmacy was bypassed by supplying the patient with the medication at the clinic. The therapist would give precise instructions of how and when to take the medication and the possibility of side-effects. By developing a personal relationship with every patient and decreasing the time spent in the clinic from an average of 4 h to 15–20 min, our drop-out rate was reduced from 42% to under 4% in a matter of 2 years. In addition, 85% of the patients followed in this clinic for more than 2 years now have normal blood pressure.

PREVALENCE OF NON-COMPLIANCE

Most physicians do not realize how significant their drop-out problem really is – they have no idea how many of their hypertensive patients do not come back.

Non-compliance rates vary widely. Most studies[2–5] have shown that about 20% of patients with symptoms do not keep their appointments and about 50% do not take their medication as directed. When patients are asymptomatic, as most hypertensive patients are, failure to keep follow-up appointments is about 50% and non-compliance with medications is in the neighbourhood of 60%.

Interesting also is the inability of the average physician to predict how many of his patients, or indeed, which patients, are not going to return. Davis's[2] survey of 132 faculty physicians and 86 fourth-year medical students who practised in the clinic of a large metropolitan hospital shows what poor predictors we really are. About 60% of those surveyed returned their views on the problem of patient compliance. In contrast to the high degree of non-compliance found in the literature, 56% of the faculty stated that almost all of their patients adhered to the prescribed medical advice; 37% said that three-quarters or more adhered. Only 7% thought that one-half or fewer of their patients complied.

The fourth-year medical students' view was more consistent with the literature. Only 22% thought that almost all of their patients adhered; 60% thought that three-quarters adhered, and 18% thought that one-half or fewer complied.

The 'drop-out' problem is not peculiar to the clinic. The private practitioner frequently does not notice that a large number of his patients fail to return for follow-up. The cavalier attitude that many physicians take regarding patients 'th mild and moderately severe hypertension is demonstrated by the recent studies of Schoenberger[6] which revealed that 55% of newly discovered hypertensive patients in the offices of cardiologists, and internists were not even given a second appointment.

IMPROVING COMPLIANCE

Regular follow-up
Routine follow-up appointments at regular intervals should be given for all hypertensive patients, whether they are on medication or not. If a patient fails to keep his appointment, he should be contacted and a new appointment made. Good follow-up is absolutely essential.

Frequency of dosage
Many studies[7–9] have demonstrated that the simpler the treatment, the more likely the patient will remain on therapy. The greatest compliance obviously follows a one-pill-a-day regimen. In this regard, the good effect of a combination of thiazides plus reserpine in the Veterans Administration studies should be emphasized[10]. The addition of a third drug, hydralazine, resulted in only a 4 mm further reduction in diastolic pressure. If such simple therapy produced these good results in men whose diastolic pressure were in the 114–129 mmHg range, it is logical to assume that this simple type of regimen would at least be as satisfactory in the male patients with less severe disease. As a matter of fact complicated regimens are rarely indicated. A recent study in an inner-city population[1] where an 8-months drop-out rate was only 3%, has demonstrated that in 70% of newly discovered hypertensive patients, the blood pressure was brought to normal by a combination tablet of reserpine plus chlorthalidone – one pill a day.

We have found several other ways to help the patient take his medication correctly. First of all it is important to change the patient's way of life as little as possible, at least at the beginning.

Pill-taking reminders
There is no doubt that the patient would benefit from giving up smoking and losing weight, in addition to taking an antihypertensive agent, but he is more likely to take his medication if this is all you ask him to do. Convenient packaging of medication also enhances pill-taking. The oral contraceptive type of packaging can surely be used for once-a-day antihypertensive therapy. When more than one medication is prescribed, the use of one of the many commercially available containers with compartments for every day of the week provides the patient with a checklist that helps him take his daily quota. Taking the medication in association

with a daily activity, i.e., once daily with breakfast, or twice daily with the morning and evening brushing of the teeth, reinforces the patient's medication schedule.

Support from physician, family, and pharmacist
Finally in this regard we all do better with at least some degree of supervision, particularly as far as taking medication is concerned. In my experience, patients are more likely to take their medication properly if the doctor (or nurse) shows a particular interest and specifically asks the patient whether he is taking his medication on schedule and whether the pills bother him in any way. The physician should also enlist the help of the spouse in this regard – as a matter of fact, the more the long-term management of the hypertensive patient can become a family affair, the better. Those patients living alone obviously present a special problem, particularly young males and the elderly. Lastly, the pharmacist can be extremely helpful in reminding the patient to take his medication and keep his appointment.

The actual writing of the prescription, warning of its possible side-effects and specifying the exact time of day that the patient should take the medication should be an integral part of the office visit. So often the prescription seems to be an afterthought, hurriedly handed to the patient as he is going out the door, with the instructions, 'Don't forget to take this'. When there is more than one prescription, the patient frequently will buy only one since 'after all, it was not that important in the first place'.

Close attention to side-effects
Failure to comply is also commonly due to drug-induced side-effects, frequently from drugs the patient does not really need. The patient is either too embarrassed to discuss the side-effects since he wants to please the physician by making a good report, or he does not realize that the side-effects are drug-related. In this regard, it should be emphasized that the more potent the antihypertensive effect, the more frequent and obnoxious are the side-effects. Patients with mild disease therefore should not be subjected to potent antihypertensive agents with the possibility of undesirable side-effects. Indeed, the objectionable side-effects may be worse than the actual disease. When patients have severe vascular disease with complications such as congestive heart failure, a cerebral vascular accident or failing vision, side-effects will readily be tolerated since the choice here is not between enjoying or not enjoying but between living or dying. In patients with mild disease (most hypertensives), however, who are truly asymptomatic – even minor side-effects are frequently not tolerated.

The patient must be told in loud and clear terms at the outset that there are a variety of drugs available, and that if one regimen is troublesome, another can be substituted. The goal of therapy is not simply the lowest blood pressure that can be obtained but *the lowest blood pressure with the fewest side-effects*. In my experience, this goal can be accomplished in 85% of patients regardless of the severity of the disease. A frank discussion with the patient emphasizing the need for mutual cooperation and free communication – that you are not only interested in lowering his blood pressure but also allowing him to enjoy a full life – will do much to start a meaningful relationship.

When a new drug is added to the regimen it is important to initiate therapy with a suboptimal dosage. For instance, methyldopa and hydralazine should be initiated in doses of 250 mg and 25 mg respectively once a day. The dose of both these drugs can then be gradually increased over a 2-week period to 1000 mg of methyldopa and 100 mg of hydralazine, each given in divided doses. Instituting therapy with either of these agents in the usually recommended dosage (i.e., methyldopa, 250 mg, four times daily and hydralazine, 25 mg, three times daily) will frequently be associated with obnoxious side-effects. Unpleasant side-effects during the first day of a new medication will 'turn the patient off' from taking this drug for ever, and has the real possibility of making him refuse all antihypertensive therapy for the rest of his life.

Importance of close patient–therapist relationship
It has been my experience, both in private practice and in the clinic, that patients (particularly those who are asymptomatic) will not remain under medical care and on medication unless they are properly motivated. Such motivation can only result from a good patient–therapist relationship. (Recent experience with an inner-city population has attested to the fact that a well-trained, understanding, sympathetic paramedical person may be substituted for the physician in this relationship.) Once this relationship has been established, time can then be spent in educating the patient rather than merely reassuring him. Education in the absence of such a relationship is worthless.

To quote Podell[11], at least a dozen studies show a positive association between patient knowledge and compliance. On the other hand, at least two dozen studies show no such relationship. The problem, as Podell states, is not whether there is an association between compliance and patient knowledge, but whether teaching patients about their illness works. In my experience the result of teaching patients is absolutely dependent on a good doctor– (or nurse)–patient relationship.

Establishing such a relationship obviously entails continuity of physician (or nurse-pharmacist) care, i.e., being followed by the same physician-nurse in the clinic or private office rather than the traditional clinic routine of a different physician each visit. In addition, it seems obvious that manifesting a sincere interest in the patient, in his blood pressure levels, specifically asking whether or not he is taking his medication, whether the medicine is bothering him in any way, whether he feels different in any way, emphasizing and re-emphasizing specific instructions and asking the patient whether he fully understands, all go a long way in developing a meaningful relationship. Simply taking the time to ask these questions frequently convinces the patient of your sincerity – that you really care. How many times have we treated our private patient in an absolutely impersonal fashion as though he were a number in the grocery store (clinic patients are frequently treated like this routinely). How many times have we made ourselves unapproachable, preventing the patient from even thinking about asking a question, by constantly looking at the clock or into the waiting room to see how many patients are left?

Let's be honest with ourselves! Physicians are not interested in, or challenged by, following apparently healthy patients, particularly patients that do not have any symptoms. Physicians are crisis-oriented and are more interested in relief of pain and solving the acute problem. The more specialized the physician's training, the less interested he is in asymptomatic 'dull' patients. The expertise of the cardiologist, as an example, has centred around the unravelling of complicated diagnostic problems or treating the patient in the emergency-crisis situation. The long-term routine care of the hypertensive patient offers no challenge.

Role of nurse specialist

Just as specially educated nurses are relied on for the routine patient care in the coronary intensive care unit, their value in the long-term follow-up of hypertensive patients should be evident. Once the hypertensive patient has been initially evaluated and placed on a therapeutic regimen by a physician and has reached a *status quo* situation, he can then ideally be followed by a nurse or health assistant working under the nurse. There is no need for the physician to examine the patient on every visit. The nurse is challenged by this assignment, and seeks to establish a meaningful relationship with the patient which then allows her to motivate the patient to take medication and remain under care for the rest of his life.

Wherever such projects have been carried out they have been successful and acceptable by the patient. The Amos Project at Fort Belvoir, the Ambulatory Care Project at the Beth Israel Hospital in Boston and the Hypertension Detection and Follow-up Program in inner-city Washington are a few examples. Utilization of the specially educated nurse and paramedical personnel goes a long way towards eliminating the over-crowding in clinics. Furthermore, patients realize that the physician and nurse team are working together to promote the optimum care possible. The effectiveness of a nurse-supervised, paramedically operated clinic in controlling blood pressure in inner-city Washington at the District of Columbia General Hospital has been alluded to above. The key to suc-cess of this programme lies in the basic assumption that the vast majority of patients with hypertension have mild or moderately severe disease and can, therefore, be readily treated, often on a regimen as simple as one pill a day. The problem is keeping the patient coming back.

With a trained nurse effectively directing the clinic in consultation with a physician and assisted by two paramedics, 30–40 patients could easily be seen per day. Doubling the paramedical personnel (ours are recruited from the community and trained by the clinic staff) could usually double the number of patients such a clinic can handle. Con-sidering the roughly eight-to-one cost ratio of physician to paramedical personnel this arrangement not only leads to substantial economic savings but also frees the doctor to carry out other duties.

Heavy reliance on specially educated nurses has also been shown to be successful in following and treating hypertensive subjects in industry. A recent project by Alderman dovetailed a screening and treatment facility at a large department store in New York City[12]. His operation was a success from every aspect. At the end of the first year the blood pressure had been brought under control in 80% of the patients; 97% of the orig-inal patients were still under treatment and the cost per patient was less than $100 per year. The union was so encouraged by the low cost, de-creased disability and time lost from work that they began to represent the programme as a 'membership benefit' and are currently supporting its expansion.

Since health care is predominantly delivered by the private prac-titioner, we are currently evaluating the role of a trained nurse in a pri-vate practice setting[13]. A specially educated nurse is currently being placed in the offices of a family practitioner in suburbia and a group of internists in Washington, DC. Her responsibilities are the recording of blood pressure on every patient and, at the discretion of the physician, either evaluating and treating the newly discovered hypertensive patient, or 'taking over' only after the physician has placed the patient on a thera-peutic regimen and the patient has reached a *status quo* situation. On a pilot basis, the Blue Shield organization has agreed to pay the patient's bill when treated by the nurse just as though he were treated by the doctor. This organization will also evaluate the control of blood pressure, the number of drop-outs, the patient's acceptance of the nurse and, most important, the impact of the nurse on the office efficiency and economy.

With the nurse taking over the long-term management of the hypertensive patients, the physician will have additional time to treat many more sick patients. It is hoped that at the end of a year the data will demonstrate an increased incidence of hypertensive patients (since blood pressure recording wiil be carried out on every patient), an increase in the number of hypertensive patients under therapy, better control of the arterial pressure and a decreased incidence of drop-outs.

Role of the pharmacist

In addition to the nurse, it is my firm belief that recruiting the pharmacist to be on the doctor-nurse team will greatly enhance compliance. In no way am I suggesting that the pharmacist take the place of the nurse or the physician, but in conjunction with them he can help educate the patient and keep him on medication and under medical care. The pharmacist is the most un-used (and probably unappreciated) person in the health delivery system. His major expertise is in the use of drugs, their modes of action and interactions and precise dosage schedules. How many times is he called upon to utilize this expertise? He really is capable of doing more than simply operating a drug store.

If the pharmacist is going to be helpful to the physician in enhancing patient compliance, the physician must 'start the ball rolling' by writing specific instructions on every prescription, not just 'as directed'. The pharmacist can then re-emphasize the number of pills, time of day, before or after eating, etc., which the physician may not have had time to do. By keeping a current drug profile on every patient, the pharmacist might well find that the patient is taking another medication (i.e., for depression, or a skin rash) which might decrease the effectiveness of, or cause possible toxicity with, the antihypertensive medication. Most patients usually go to the same pharmacy as a matter of convenience – at work or at home. Relating with the same pharmacist and having the pharmacist relate with the physician simply adds one more member to the health delivery team all programmed to help the patient take his medication correctly and stay under medical care for the rest of his life.

SUMMARY

Although the attack on the patient non-compliance may differ according to the population and location, several general principles apply to all:

1 People, whether in Africa or America, Alaska, Hawaii, very much respond to being treated humanely and with dignity.
2 The more the patient knows about his disease and its complications,

the more readily he is going to comply.

Although an efficient appointment system, providing services conveniently for the patient, keeping therapy simple, keeping the cost of medication and laboratory tests at a minimum all are capable of enhancing compliance, they are not substitutes for a meaningful doctor–patient or nurse–patient relationship. The asymptomatic patient, educated or uneducated, black or white, is not going to remain on therapy and under medical care unless he is positively motivated, and such motivation can only stem from a meaningful personal therapist–patient relationship.

References

1 Finnerty, F. A., Jr., Mattie, E. C. and Finnerty, F. A., III. (1973). Hypertension in the inner city. I. Analysis of clinic drop-outs. *Circulation*, **47**, 73
2 Davis, M. S. (1966). Varations in patients' compliance with doctor's orders: analysis of congruence between survey responses and results of empirical investigations. *J. Med. Educ.*, **41**, 1037
3 McKinlay, J. B. (1972) Some approaches and problems in the study of the use of services – an overview. *J. Health Soc. Behav.*, **13**, 115
4 Gillum, R. F. and Barsky, A. J. (1974). Diagnosis and management of patient non-compliance. *J. Am. Med. Assoc.*, **228**, 1563
5 Blackwell, B. (1973). Patient compliance. *N. Engl. J. Med.*, **289**, 249
6 Schoenberger, J. A., Stamler, J., Shekelle, R. B. and Shekelle, S. (1972). Current status of hypertension control in the industrial population. *J. Am. Med. Assoc.*, **222**, 559
7 Francis, V., Korsch, B. M and Morris, M. J. (1969). Gaps in doctor–patient communications. Patients' response to medical advice. *N. Engl. J. Med.*, **280**, 535
8 Marston, M. V. (1970). Compliance with medical regimens: A review of the literature. *Nurs. Res.*, **19**, 312
9 Finnerty, F. A., Jr. (1974). The hypertension problem. What we can do about it. *Circulation*, **48**, 681
10 Veterans Administration Cooperative Study Group on Antihypertensive Agents: effects of treatment on morbidity in hypertension. II. Results in patients with diastolic blood pressure averaging 90 through 114 mmHg. (1970). *J. Am. Med. Assoc.*, **213**, 1143
11 Podell, R. N. (1975) *Physician's Guide to Compliance in Hypertension.* (Merck Sharp & Dohme)
12 Alderman, M. H. and Schoenbaum, E. E. (1975). Detection and treatment of hypertension at the work site. *N. Engl. J. Med.*, **293**, 65
13 Finnerty, F. A., Jr. (1975). The nurses' role in treating hypertension. *N. Engl. J. Med.*, **293**, 93

Index